Teen Health Series

Learning Disabilities Information For Teens, Second Edition

Learning Disabilities Information For Teens, Second Edition

Health Tips About Academic Skills
Disorders And Other Disabilities
That Affect Learning

Including Information About Common Signs
Of Learning Disabilities, School Issues, Learning To Live
With A Learning Disability, And Other Related Issues

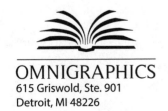

OMNIGRAPHICS
615 Griswold, Ste. 901
Detroit, MI 48226

Bibliographic Note
Because this page cannot legibly accommodate all the copyright notices, the Bibliographic Note portion of the Preface constitutes an extension of the copyright notice.

* * *

Omnigraphics
a part of Relevant Information
Keith Jones, *Managing Editor*

* * *

Library of Congress Cataloging-in-Publication Data

Names: Omnigraphics, Inc.

Title: Learning disabilities information for teens: health tips about academic skills disorders and other disabilities that affect learning including information about common signs of learning disabilities, school issues, learning to live with a learning disability, and other related issues.

Description: Second edition. | Detroit, MI: Omnigraphics, [2017] | Series: Teen health series | Includes bibliographical references and index. | Audience: Grade 9 to 12.

Identifiers: LCCN 2016056339 (print) | LCCN 2016058190 (ebook) | ISBN 9780780814721 (hardcover: alk. paper) | ISBN 9780780814714 (ebook) | ISBN 9780780814714 (eBook)

Subjects: LCSH: Learning disabilities--Health aspects.

Classification: LCC RJ496.L4 L434 2017 (print) | LCC RJ496.L4 (ebook) | DDC 618.92/85889--dc23

LC record available at https://lccn.loc.gov/2016056339

Table Of Contents

Part Four: Other Disabilities And Chronic Conditions That Affect Learning

Part Five: Academic Issues

Part Six: Living With A Learning Disability

Preface

About This Book

In the United States, nearly 6.5 million children and youth ages 3–21 currently receive special education services for learning disabilities, such as dyslexia, dyscalculia, and other disorders that affect language development, motor control, attention, and behavior. It is important to understand how students with learning disabilities can be helped. According to the 2016 *Building a Grad Nation Data Brief*, students without identified disabilities graduated at a rate of 84.8 percent, compared with just 63.1 percent of students with disabilities—a gap of more than 21 percentage points. In addition 33 states graduate less than 70 percent of their students with disabilities Identifying and addressing problems as early as possible enables students to develop the skills and coping strategies needed to succeed in school and beyond.

Learning Disabilities Information For Teens, Second Edition, describes the different kinds of learning disabilities and their common signs, causes, and diagnostic procedures. It also discusses how other disabilities and chronic conditions can affect learning. Information on academic issues, such as homework, study habits, and assistive technology, is included along with coping tips and facts about laws designed to protect the rights of people with learning disabilities. Suggestions for additional reading and a directory of organizations able to provide help and further information are also included.

How To Use This Book

This book is divided into parts and chapters. Parts focus on broad areas of interest; chapters are devoted to single topics within a part.

Part I: Learning Disabilities: An Overview defines learning disabilities, describes common signs, and discusses current myths and misconceptions about learning disabilities. Information on causes and diagnosing learning disabilities is also provided.

Part II: Types Of Learning Disabilities describes the three categories of learning disabilities—academic skills disorders, developmental speech and language disorders, and other disorders that include impaired sensory and motor skills and information processing issues. The often-overlooked problems faced by gifted students with learning disabilities are also discussed.

Part III: Co-Occurring Disorders takes a look at the types of problems that often accompany learning disabilities and complicate their treatment, including attention deficit hyperactivity disorder (ADHD), substance abuse, and bipolar disorder.

Part IV: Other Disabilities And Chronic Conditions That Affect Learning provides information on medical conditions and physical challenges that can affect a student's ability to learn either by interrupting the educational process or by affecting the ways in which the brain processes information. These include cancer treatment aphasia, cerebral palsy, epilepsy, autism, Down syndrome, Tourette syndrome, abusive head trauma, XYY syndrome, triple-X syndrome, Klinefelter syndrome, and Turner syndrome.

Part V: Academic Issues provides facts about understanding and accessing different school options. It explains how to evaluate a learning disability, why it is important, and how to develop an Individualized Education Plan (IEP). It provides practical suggestions for areas that may be especially challenging, including doing homework, improving study skills, and providing effective academic instruction for children with ADHD. It also provides information on available assistive technology, explains career development options, and offers tips about transition planning and evaluating educational options after high school.

Part VI: Living With A Learning Disability offers help to students in areas where they may face challenges outside of the classroom, self-esteem, self-advocacy, and social skills. Commonly encountered problems, such as bullying, coping with sibling issues, barriers to participation, and employment discrimination, are also discussed.

Part VII: Learning Disabilities And Your Legal Rights provides information on the laws that protect people with learning disabilities. These include the Individuals with Disabilities Education Act (IDEA), Section 504 of the Rehabilitation Act, and the Americans with Disabilities Act (ADA).

Part VIII: If You Need More Information provides a directory of organizations able to provide additional help or support, and a list of selected online apps and games that can assist those with learning disabilities.

Bibliographic Note

This volume contains documents and excerpts from publications issued by the following U.S. government agencies: Administration for Children and Families (ACF); Center for Parent Information and Resources (CPIR); Centers for Disease Control and Prevention

(CDC); Corporation for National and Community Service (CNCS); *Eunice Kennedy Shriver* National Institute of Child Health and Human Development (NICHD); Genetic and Rare Diseases Information Center (GARD); Genetics Home Reference (GHR); Job Corps; National Cancer Institute (NCI); National Center on Birth Defects and Developmental Disabilities (NCBDDD); National Institute of Diabetes and Digestive and Kidney Diseases (NIDDK); National Institute of Mental Health (NIMH); National Institute of Neurological Disorders and Stroke (NINDS); National Institute on Deafness and Other Communication Disorders (NIDCD); Office of Disability Employment Policy (ODEP); Office of Special Education Programs (OSEP); Substance Abuse and Mental Health Services Administration (SAMHSA); U.S. Department of Education (ED); U.S. Department of Health and Human Services (HHS); U.S. Department of Justice (DOJ); U.S. Department of Labor (DOL); U.S. Drug Enforcement Administration (DEA); U.S. Environmental Protection Agency (EPA); and U.S. Senate Committee on Health, Education, Labor, and Pensions (HELP).

In addition, this volume contains copyrighted documents from the following organizations:

Learning Disabilities Association of America (LDA)
The Nemours Foundation
Understood.org USA LLC

It may also contain original material produced by Omnigraphics and reviewed by medical consultants.

The photograph on the front cover is © Alejandro Rivera/iStock.

Medical Review

Omnigraphics contracts with a team of qualified, senior medical professionals who serve as medical consultants for the *Teen Health Series*. As necessary, medical consultants review reprinted and originally written material for currency and accuracy. Citations including the phrase, Reviewed (month, year)" indicate material reviewed by this team. Medical consultation services are provided to the *Teen Health Series* editors by:

Dr. Senthil Selvan, MBBS, DCH, MD
Dr. K. Sivanandham, MBBS, DCH, MS (Research), PhD

About The *Teen Health Series*

At the request of librarians serving today's young adults, the *Teen Health Series* was developed as a specially focused set of volumes within Omnigraphics' *Health Reference Series*. Each volume deals comprehensively with a topic selected according to the needs and interests of people in middle school and high school. Teens seeking preventive guidance, information about disease warning signs, medical statistics, and risk factors for health problems will find answers to their questions in the *Teen Health Series*. The *Series*, however, is not intended to serve as a tool for diagnosing illness, in prescribing treatments, or as a substitute for the physician/patient relationship. All people concerned about medical symptoms or the possibility of disease are encouraged to seek professional care from an appropriate health care provider.

If there is a topic you would like to see addressed in a future volume of the *Teen Health Series*, please write to:

Editor
Teen Health Series
Omnigraphics
615 Griswold, Ste. 901
Detroit, MI 48226

A Note About Spelling And Style

Teen Health Series editors use *Stedman's Medical Dictionary* as an authority for questions related to the spelling of medical terms and the *Chicago Manual of Style* for questions related to grammatical structures, punctuation, and other editorial concerns. Consistent adherence is not always possible, however, because the individual volumes within the *Series* include many documents from a wide variety of different producers and copyright holders, and the editor's primary goal is to present material from each source as accurately as is possible following the terms specified by each document's producer. This sometimes means that information in different chapters or sections may follow other guidelines and alternate spelling authorities.

Part One
Learning Disabilities: An Overview

Chapter 1
What Is A Learning Disability?

Learning disabilities are conditions that affect how a person learns to read, write, speak, and calculate numbers. They are caused by differences in brain structure and affect the way a person's brain processes information.

Learning disabilities are usually discovered after a child begins attending school and has difficulties in one or more subjects that do not improve over time. A person can have more than one learning disability. Learning disabilities can last a person's entire life, but they may be alleviated with the right educational supports.

> A learning disability is not an indication of a person's intelligence. Also, learning disabilities are not the same as learning problems due to intellectual and developmental disabilities, or emotional, vision, hearing, or motor skills problems.

Some of the most common learning disabilities include the following:

- **Dyslexia.** This condition causes problems with language skills, particularly reading. People with dyslexia may have difficulty spelling, understanding sentences, and recognizing words they already know.

- **Dysgraphia.** People with dysgraphia have problems with their handwriting. They may have problems forming letters, writing within a defined space, and writing down their thoughts.

About This Chapter: This chapter includes text excerpted from "Learning Disabilities," *Eunice Kennedy Shriver National Institute of Child Health and Human Development* (NICHD), December 5, 2012. Reviewed December 2016.

- **Dyscalculia.** People with this math learning disability may have difficulty understanding arithmetic concepts and doing such tasks as addition, multiplication, and measuring.

- **Dyspraxia.** This condition, also termed sensory integration disorder, involves problems with motor coordination that lead to poor balance and clumsiness. Poor hand-eye coordination also causes difficulty with fine motor tasks such as putting puzzles together and coloring within the lines.

- **Apraxia of speech.** Sometimes called verbal apraxia, this disorder involves problems with speaking. People with this disorder have trouble saying what they want to say correctly and consistently.

- **Central auditory processing disorder.** People with this condition have trouble understanding and remembering language-related tasks. They have difficulty explaining things, understanding jokes, and following directions. They confuse words and are easily distracted.

- **Nonverbal learning disorders.** People with these conditions have strong verbal skills but great difficulty understanding facial expression and body language. In addition, they are physically clumsy and have trouble generalizing and following multistep directions.

- **Visual perceptual/visual motor deficit.** People with this condition mix up letters; they might confuse "m" and "w" or "d" and "b," for example. They may also lose their place while reading, copy inaccurately, write messily, and cut paper clumsily.

- **Aphasia.** Aphasia, also called dysphasia, is a language disorder. A person with this disorder has difficulty understanding spoken language, poor reading comprehension, trouble with writing, and great difficulty finding words to express thoughts and feelings. Aphasia occurs when the language areas of the brain are damaged. In adults, it often is caused by stroke, but children may get aphasia from a brain tumor, head injury, or brain infection.

How Many People Are Affected / At Risk For Learning Disabilities?

There is a wide range in estimates of the number of people affected by learning disabilities and disorders. Some of the variation results from differences in requirements for diagnosis in different states.

Some reports estimate that as many as 15 percent to 20 percent of Americans are affected by learning disabilities and disorders. In contrast, a major national study found that approximately

5 percent of children in the United States had learning disabilities. It also found that approximately 4 percent had both a learning disability and attention deficit hyperactivity disorder (ADHD).

How Are Learning Disabilities Diagnosed?

Learning disabilities are often identified when a child begins to attend school. Educators may use a process called "response to intervention" (RTI) to help identify children with learning disabilities. Specialized testing is required to make a clear diagnosis, however.

RTI

RTI usually involves the following:

- Monitoring all students' progress closely to identify possible learning problems.
- Providing a child identified as having problems with help on different levels, or tiers.
- Moving this youngster through the tiers as appropriate, increasing educational assistance if the child does not show progress.

Students who are struggling in school can also have individual evaluations. An evaluation can:

- Identify whether a child has a learning disability.
- Determine a child's eligibility under federal law for special education services.
- Help construct an Individualized Education Plan (IEP) that outlines supports for a youngster who qualifies for special education services.
- Establish a benchmark for measuring the child's educational progress

A full evaluation for a learning disability includes the following:

- A medical examination, including a neurological exam, to identify or rule out other possible causes of the child's difficulties, including emotional disorders, intellectual and developmental disabilities, and brain diseases.
- Exploration of the youngster's developmental, social, and school performance.
- A discussion of family history.
- Academic achievement testing and psychological assessment.

Usually, several specialists work as a team to perform an evaluation. The team may include a psychologist, special education expert, and speech-language pathologist (SLP). Many schools also have reading specialists on staff who can help diagnosis a reading disability.

Role Of School Psychologists

School psychologists are trained in both education and psychology. They can help to identify students with learning disabilities and can diagnose the learning disability. They can also help the student with the disability, parents, and teachers come up with plans that improve learning.

Role Of SLPs

All SLPs are trained in diagnosing and treating speech- and language-related disorders. A SLP can provide a complete language evaluation as well as an assessment of the child's ability to organize his or her thoughts and possessions. The SLP may evaluate various age-appropriate learning-related skills in the child, such as understanding directions, manipulating sounds, and reading and writing.

Is There A Cure For Learning Disabilities?

Learning disabilities have no cure, but early intervention can provide tools and strategies to lessen their effects. People with learning disabilities can be successful in school and work and in their personal lives.

What Are The Treatments For Learning Disabilities?

People with learning disabilities and disorders can learn strategies for coping with their disabilities. Getting help earlier increases the likelihood for success in school and later in life. If learning disabilities remain untreated, a child may begin to feel frustrated with schoolwork, which can lead to low self-esteem, depression, and other problems.

Usually, experts work to help a child learn skills by building on the child's strengths and developing ways to compensate for the child's weaknesses. Interventions vary depending on the nature and extent of the disability.

Special Education Services

Children diagnosed with learning and other disabilities can qualify for special educational services. The Individuals with Disabilities Education Improvement Act (IDEA) requires that the public school system provide free special education supports to children with disabilities.

In most states, each child is entitled to these services beginning when he or she is 3 years old and extending through high school or until age 21, whichever comes first. The specific rules of IDEA for each state are available from the National Early Childhood Technical Assistance Center.

IDEA states that children must be taught in the least restrictive environments appropriate for them. This means the teaching environment should be designed to meet a child's specific needs and skills and should minimize restrictions on the youngster's access to typical learning experiences.

IEPs

A child who qualifies for special education services should receive his or her own IEP. This personalized and written education plan:

- Lists individualized goals for the child

- Specifies the plan for services the youngster will receive

- Lists the specialists who will work with the child

Qualifying For Special Education

To qualify for special education services, a child must be evaluated by the school system and meet specific criteria outlined in federal and state guidelines. To learn how to have a child assessed for special services, parents and caregivers can contact a local school principal or special education coordinator.

Interventions For Specific Learning Disabilities

Below are just a few examples of ways educators help children with specific learning disabilities.

Dyslexia

- **Special teaching techniques.** These can include helping a child learn through multisensory experiences and by providing immediate feedback to strengthen a child's ability to recognize words.

- **Classroom modifications.** For example, teachers can give students with dyslexia extra time to finish tasks and provide taped tests that allow the child to hear the questions instead of reading them.

- **Use of technology.** Children with dyslexia may benefit from listening to books on tape or using word-processing programs with spell-check features.

Dysgraphia

- **Special tools.** Teachers can offer oral exams, provide a note-taker, and/or allow the child to videotape reports instead of writing them.

- **Use of technology.** A child with dysgraphia can be taught to use word-processing programs or an audio recorder instead of writing by hand.

- **Other ways of reducing the need for writing.** Teachers can provide notes, outlines, and preprinted study sheets.

Dyscalculia

- **Visual techniques.** For example, teachers can draw pictures of word problems and show the student how to use colored pencils to differentiate parts of problems.

- **Use of memory aids.** Rhymes and music are among the techniques that can be used to help a child remember math concepts.

- **Use of computers.** A child with dyscalculia can use a computer for drills and practice.

Dyspraxia

- **Quiet learning environment.** To help a child deal with sensitivity to noise and distractions, educators can provide the youngster with a quiet place for tests, silent reading, and other tasks that require concentration.

- **Alerting the child in advance.** For example, a child who is sensitive to noise may benefit from knowing in advance about such events as fire drills and assemblies.

- **Occupational therapy.** Exercises that focus on the tasks of daily living can help a child with poor coordination.

Other Treatments

A child with a learning disability may struggle with low self-esteem, frustration, and other problems. Mental health professionals can help the youngster understand these feelings, develop coping tools, and build healthy relationships.

Children with learning disabilities sometimes have other conditions such as ADHD. These conditions require their own treatments, which may include therapy and medications.

Are There Disorders Or Conditions Associated With Learning Disabilities?

Children with learning disabilities may be at greater risk for certain conditions than other youngsters.

One condition found more frequently among children with learning disabilities is ADHD. A child with ADHD may be very active and impulsive and get distracted easily. ADHD affects about 1 out of 3 children with learning disorders.

Children with disabilities also may develop depression, anxiety, and behavior problems.

Treating conditions associated with a learning disability can help a child feel better over-all and become more focused on schoolwork. Treatments may include psychotherapy and medications.

Chapter 2
Myths And Misconceptions About Learning Disabilities

The adoption and acceptance of long standing "myths" and "misconceptions" regarding individuals with learning and attention disabilities continues to fuel prejudicial views, erect attitudinal barriers, and create social stigmas that can have devastating long-term results— emotionally and educationally. Because learning and attention disabilities are not always readily obvious to others, these individuals often get labeled as "stupid," "lazy," "space cadet," "dumb," and other such derogatory terms. These terms only serve to exacerbate the negative self-image that many youth with these disabilities already have about themselves.

Dispelling these myths and misconceptions requires ongoing education and training for the general public as well as service providers, family members, and the student with the disability.

Dispelling The Myths And Misconceptions About Learning Disabilities (LD)

Myth: Individuals with LD have limited potential.

Truth: Individuals with LD conduct successful and fulfilling lives just as individuals without disabilities do. Greater success is achieved when these individuals are appropriately accommodated or have developed effective compensatory strategies.

Myth: LD is just a polite way to refer to lower overall intelligence and abilities.

Truth: Inherent within the definition of LD is a discrepancy between demonstrated intelligence and specific functioning. It is possible for a student to be both gifted and learning disabled at the same time.

About This Chapter: This chapter includes text excerpted from "Myths And Misconceptions," Job Corps, U.S. Department of Labor (DOL), August 23, 2014.

Myth: People with LD are lazy.

Truth: If an individual with a LD has experienced repeated failures, particularly educationally or socially, they often shut down and believe it hurts less to not try than it does to try and fail. The individual may feel he/she has no control over what happens to her/him which is known as learned helplessness. Small doses of success are the best antidote to learned helplessness.

> Having a learning disability does not mean that you are slow or dumb. It means that your brain is "wired" a bit differently, so that you learn differently from most other kids.
>
> *(Source: "Learning Disabilities And ADHD," girlshealth.gov, Office on Women's Health (OWH).)*

Myth: Given proper instruction, individuals with LD can grow out of it.

Truth: Although individuals with LD can and do acquire improved skills, the LD themselves are not cured in the process. Some types of LD can be successfully and permanently remediated but others are thought to be lifelong and may require the acquisition and use of compensatory strategies or accommodations throughout the individual's life span.

Myth: Accommodations provided to students with LD, particularly during testing situations, gives them an unfair advantage over students without disabilities.

Truth: An accommodation does not tip the scales in the student's favor; it merely levels the playing field. Accommodations provide access to the information thus giving the student with a disability a means to demonstrate his/her knowledge, skills, and abilities. Without modifications, common forms of instruction and examination often inadvertently reflect a student's disability rather than the subject at hand. For example, a student who has a writing disability would be greatly impaired during a written essay exam even though he/she was skilled in the art and mechanics of writing an essay. The use of a word processor allows this student to demonstrate his/her knowledge rather than be judged by the limitations his handwriting difficulties imposed.

Myth: Accommodating the needs of a student with LD means watering down course and program requirements.

Truth: Teaching a student with special learning needs does not mean "less." It may, however, mean "different." The instructional goal should be to find ways to work around the area of deficit and still impart the same body of information and sets of skills.

Myth: Students with LD do not have to work any harder than other students.

Truth: Most students with LD do have to work harder than the average student to achieve success. However, the "silver lining" for those who are willing to put in the extra effort is that being a hard worker is a highly valued characteristic in the work world.

Dispelling The Myths And Misconceptions About Attention Deficit Hyperactivity Disorder (ADHD)

Myth: ADHD does not really exist. It is simply the latest excuse for parents who do not discipline their children.

Truth: Scientific research tells us ADHD is a biologically based disorder that includes distractibility, impulsiveness, and sometimes hyperactivity. Before a student is diagnosed with ADHD, other possible causes of his/her behavior are ruled out.

Myth: Medication can cure students with ADHD.

Truth: Medicine cannot cure ADHD but can sometimes temporarily moderate its effects. Certain stimulant medications are effective in the majority of the individuals who take it, providing an immediate short-term increase in attention, control, concentration, and goal-directed effort. Medication may also reduce disruptive behaviors, aggression, and hyperactivity.

Myth: Individuals with ADHD will outgrow it.

Truth: ADHD is a lifelong condition although it manifests itself differently dependent upon the age of the individual. Some individuals

1. experience a lessening of ADHD symptoms with age,

2. develop effective compensatory strategies that make it appear as if the ADHD has gone away, or

3. manage the symptoms of the disorder with medication.

Myth: Individuals who can focus their attention in some areas (i.e., video games, etc.) cannot have ADHD.

Truth: ADHD is a neurological difference that makes it very difficult to attend to things that are not interesting to the person involved or that require sustained mental effort. Yet this person can sit for hours and play video games or participate in other activities of interest. This type of focus is known as hyperfocus.

Lots of things about having ADHD can be challenging—especially added on top of the usual stress a teen faces. But there are so many things you can do to feel better. Find ways to use your skills, relax, and connect with other people.

(Source: "Learning Disabilities And ADHD," girlshealth.gov.)

Chapter 3
What Are Some Common Signs Of Learning Disabilities?

What Are The Indicators Of Learning Disabilities?

Many children have difficulty with reading, writing, or other learning-related tasks at some point, but this does not mean they have learning disabilities. A child with a learning disability often has several related signs, and these persist over time. The signs of learning disabilities vary from person to person. Common signs that a person may have learning disabilities include the following:

- difficulty with reading and/or writing

- problems with math skills

- difficulty remembering

- problems paying attention

- trouble following directions

- poor coordination

- difficulty with concepts related to time

- problems staying organized

A child with a learning disability also may exhibit one or more of the following:

- impetuous behavior

About This Chapter: This chapter includes text excerpted from "Learning Disabilities," *Eunice Kennedy Shriver* National Institute of Child Health and Human Development (NICHD), December 5, 2012. Reviewed December 2016.

- inappropriate responses in school or social situations

- difficulty staying on task (easily distracted)

- difficulty finding the right way to say something

- inconsistent school performance

- immature way of speaking

- difficulty listening well

- problems dealing with new things in life

- problems understanding words or concepts

These signs alone are not enough to determine that a person has a learning disability. A professional assessment is necessary to diagnose a learning disability.

Each learning disability has its own signs. Also, not every person with a particular disability will have all of the signs of that disability.

Children being taught in a second language that they are learning sometimes act in ways that are similar to the behaviors of someone with a learning disability. For this reason, learning disability assessment must take into account whether a student is bilingual or a second language learner.

Below are some common learning disabilities and the signs associated with them:

- Dyslexia

- Dysgraphia

- Dyscalculia

- Dyspraxia

Dyslexia

People with dyslexia usually have trouble making the connections between letters and sounds and with spelling and recognizing words.

People with dyslexia often show other signs of the condition. These may include:

- failure to fully understand what others are saying

- difficulty organizing written and spoken language

- delayed ability to speak

- poor self-expression (for example, saying "thing" or "stuff" for words not recalled)

- difficulty learning new vocabulary, either through reading or hearing

- trouble learning foreign languages

- slowness in learning songs and rhymes

- slow reading as well as giving up on longer reading tasks

- difficulty understanding questions and following directions

- poor spelling

- difficulty recalling numbers in sequence (for example, telephone numbers and addresses)

- trouble distinguishing left from right

Dysgraphia

Dysgraphia is characterized by problems with writing. This disorder may cause a child to be tense and awkward when holding a pen or pencil, even to the extent of contorting his or her body. A child with very poor handwriting that he or she does not outgrow may have dysgraphia.

Other signs of this condition may include:

- a strong dislike of writing and/or drawing

- problems with grammar

- trouble writing down ideas

- a quick loss of energy and interest while writing

- trouble writing down thoughts in a logical sequence

- saying words out loud while writing

- leaving words unfinished or omitting them when writing sentences

Dyscalculia

Signs of this disability include problems understanding basic arithmetic concepts, such as fractions, number lines, and positive and negative numbers.

Other symptoms may include:

- difficulty with math-related word problems

- trouble making change in cash transactions

- messiness in putting math problems on paper

- trouble recognizing logical information sequences (for example, steps in math problems)

- trouble with understanding the time sequence of events

- difficulty with verbally describing math processes

Dyspraxia

A person with dyspraxia has problems with motor tasks, such as hand-eye coordination, that can interfere with learning.

Some other symptoms of this condition include:

- problems organizing oneself and one's things

- breaking things

- trouble with tasks that require hand-eye coordination, such as coloring within the lines, assembling puzzles, and cutting precisely

- poor balance

- sensitivity to loud and/or repetitive noises, such as the ticking of a clock

- sensitivity to touch, including irritation over bothersome-feeling clothing

Chapter 4

What Causes Learning Disabilities?

The Brain And Learning Disabilities

Researchers do not know exactly what causes learning disabilities, but they appear to be related to differences in brain structure. These differences are present from birth and often are inherited. To improve understanding of learning disabilities, researchers at the *Eunice Kennedy Shriver* National Institute of Child Health and Human Development (NICHD) and elsewhere are studying areas of the brain and how they function. Scientists have found that learning disabilities are related to areas of the brain that deal with language and have used imaging studies to show that the brain of a dyslexic person develops and functions differently from a typical brain.

Alcohol can cause alterations in the structure and function of the developing brain, which continues to mature into a person's mid 20s, and it may have consequences reaching far beyond adolescence.

In adolescence, brain development is characterized by dramatic changes to the brain's structure, neuron connectivity (i.e., "wiring"), and physiology. These changes in the brain affect everything from emerging sexuality to emotionality and judgment.

(Source: "Alcohol And The Developing Brain," Substance Abuse and Mental Health Services Administration (SAMHSA).)

About This Chapter: Text under the heading "The Brain And Learning Disabilities" is excerpted from "Learning Disabilities: What Causes Learning Disabilities?" *Eunice Kennedy Shriver* National Institute of Child Health and Human Development (NICHD), December 5, 2012. Reviewed December 2016; Text under the heading "Understanding Dyslexia" is excerpted from "Understanding Dyslexia: The Intersection Of Scientific Research And Education," U.S. Senate Committee on Health, Education, Labor and Pensions (HELP), May 10, 2016.

Sometimes, factors that affect a developing fetus, such as alcohol or drug use, can lead to a learning disability. Other factors in an infant's environment may play a role as well. These can include poor nutrition and exposure to toxins such as lead in water or paint. In addition, children who do not receive the support necessary to promote their intellectual development early on may show signs of learning disabilities once they start school.

Sometimes a person may develop a learning disability later in life. Possible causes in such a case include dementia or a traumatic brain injury (TBI).

Fetal Alcohol Spectrum Disorders (FASDs) As A Cause Of Learning Disabilities

FASDs are a group of conditions that can occur in a person whose mother drank alcohol during pregnancy. These effects can include physical problems and problems with behavior and learning. Often, a person with an FASD has a mix of these problems. These conditions can affect each person in different ways, and can range from mild to severe.

A person with an FASD might have:

- poor coordination
- hyperactive behavior
- difficulty with attention
- poor memory
- difficulty in school (especially with math)
- learning disabilities
- speech and language delays
- intellectual disability or low IQ
- poor reasoning and judgment skills
- vision or hearing problems

(Source: "Fetal Alcohol Spectrum Disorders (FASDs): Facts About FASDs," Centers for Disease Control and Prevention (CDC).)

Understanding Dyslexia

Brain Imaging Technology: Advances In Understanding The Brain Bases For Reading And Dyslexia

The ability for scientists to use brain imaging technology to noninvasively study the brain's structure and function has resulted in tremendous advances to the understanding of the human brain, how it processes sensation, how it learns, how it remembers, and how it builds knowledge. Neuroscientists have been able to produce maps of brain regions underlying cognition and, importantly, skills that are uniquely human, such as reading. Reading, a cultural invention that allows us to represent speech in symbolic form, involves a coordination of the brain's language areas with the visual and auditory systems.

What researchers have learned is that the process of learning to read changes the brain's structure and function. People who never had the opportunity to learn to read manifest a different pattern of brain activity and have differences in brain anatomy compared to those who do learn to read.

Research also indicates that the brain needs to make some adjustments when becoming a reader, not only re-allocating brain functions from processing common objects to processing letters and words, but also adapting new rules. So while it is OK for objects, such as a chair, to be recognizable as the same object when it is viewed from the right or from the left, this is not OK for mirror letters such as p and q, and b and d. While these may look like the same object with mirror-reversal to a beginning reader (who will confuse them), successful reading acquisition requires that they become recognized as representing distinctly different letters.

Brain imaging technology has also heightened our understanding of dyslexia. Since the first implementation of functional magnetic resonance imaging (MRI) to study dyslexia in 1996, the field has grown rapidly and made significant contributions to the science of dyslexia. While researchers had already been using MRI to scrutinize brain structural differences in dyslexia, functional MRI has allowed researchers to visualize brain activity in groups of people with and without dyslexia.

Some of the same brain areas that are compromised for reading are also underactive when children with dyslexia solve arithmetic tasks, highlighting the far-reaching consequences of dyslexia and their complex connection to other forms of learning disabilities.

Together, brain imaging research has become an important tool for understanding reading and is a leading contributor in addressing the multitude of theories that have been proposed to explain dyslexia.

The Intersection Of Scientific Research And Education

While researchers are careful to assess what is directly causing the reading problems and to distinguish these brain differences from those that are a consequence or a byproduct of whatever is causing the dyslexia, it has become clear that children who eventually have dyslexia are likely to exhibit early signs of brain differences, much like specific behavioral measures in young children are lower for those who eventually go on to have dyslexia. This is not surprising given the brain–behavioral relationships and the fact that dyslexia is heritable. Scientific evidence supports genetic involvement, and a connection between dyslexia-associated genes and differences in brain activity.

A family history of dyslexia can be very predictive of children at risk for reading difficulties and, together with early behavioral measures of skills known to predict later reading outcome (such as phonemic awareness and letter naming), can be used to signal that a child is at risk for difficulties in learning to read.

Chapter 5

How Are Learning Disabilities Diagnosed?

Diagnosing learning disabilities (LDs) is difficult because LDs show up differently in different people and a learning disability in one area may be masked by accelerated ability in another. For instance, a child who has dyscalculia may not know how to add two numbers, but may write at a much higher grade level, leading teachers to think she is just being lazy about turning in her math homework.

Diagnosing Learning Disabilities In School-Aged Children And Adolescents

Learning disabilities often become evident when a child starts school. Teachers and other school professionals may identify students with suspected learning disabilities as they monitor the students' progress and their response to educational assistance. This is called the response to intervention (RTI) process. Parents may also bring their concerns about LDs in their children to the attention of school professionals.

If a student is suspected of having learning disabilities, further testing and evaluation will be needed.

The Individuals with Disabilities Education Act (IDEA) sets out clear rules and regulations on the process for evaluating children suspected of having LDs, so that students with LDs can take advantage of Individualized Education Plans (IEPs) when warranted. Under IDEA, an evaluation must be "full and individual" meaning it needs to be comprehensive in scope but tailored to the student as a distinct individual. Tests must be given in the language and at the level that the student understands best. Tests must investigate all the skills where the

"How Are Learning Disabilities Diagnosed?" © 2017 Omnigraphics. Reviewed June 2016.

student has difficulty. The results must give relevant information to make informed decisions on the next steps in the student's educational plan.

What Does It Mean

The Individuals with Disabilities Education Act (IDEA) is a law ensuring services to children with disabilities throughout the nation. IDEA governs how states and public agencies provide early intervention, special education and related services to eligible infants, toddlers, children and youth with disabilities.

The IEP creates an opportunity for teachers, parents, school administrators, related services personnel, and students (when appropriate) to work together to improve educational results for children with disabilities. The IEP is the cornerstone of a quality education for each child with a disability.

(Sources: "Building The Legacy: Idea 2004," U.S. Department of Education (ED); "A Guide To The Individualized Education Program," U.S. Department of Education (ED).)

In addition, the school staff must create an evaluation plan that informs the parents of all tests, observations, records they plan to use in the evaluation as well as providing the names of all evaluators.

The evaluation may include:

- **A physical examination** that looks for physical causes of LD such as vision, hearing, movement, or other health issues.

- **A psychological evaluation** to examine the student's emotional health and social skills, and determine how the student learns best.

- **Interviews** with the student, parents, and teachers to learn more about the student's academic history, behavior in and out of school, and other information that can help the evaluators with their diagnosis.

- **Behavioral assessment** is often accomplished using questionnaires filled out by teachers and parents about how the student interacts with the world in both normal and unusual situations.

- **Observation of the student** by teachers, the school psychologist, reading specialist, speech-language pathologist, and other educational professionals.

- **Standardized tests** that are selected by educational professionals based on the student's areas of strengths and weaknesses. These tests can test general ability or specific skills.

- *Intelligence and achievement tests* are used to measure the student's intellectual potential, what he or she knows and can do, and areas of the student's strengths and weaknesses. There are a variety of standard intelligence and achievement tests geared to a person's age. The evaluators then use the results of these tests to focus on what further testing needs to done.

- *Tests for reading, writing, and math* can include those that measure reading comprehension to determine the grade level at which a student should be taught; essential reading skills; oral reading (can the student read a passage aloud then answer questions on it?); pronunciation; general math skills.

- *Tests for language, motor, and processing skills* look at issues that affect a student's learning skills. Results of this type of test may suggest problems with perception, memory, planning, motor skills, attention, and comprehension of both written and spoken communications.

- **Other information already on file** including report cards and state test scores.

Based on the results of the evaluation, the school's IEP administrator will work with the student's teachers and family to draw up a plan of study to accommodate the student's LDs and determine strategies for effective learning and living.

Diagnosing Learning Disabilities In Adults

An adult may suspect he or she has a learning disability if there are problems at work or school, such as trouble with reading, understanding charts, communicating effectively, or staying on task. There may be problems with everyday tasks including reading the newspaper, balancing the checkbook, or making decisions. Likewise, if an adult has struggled to learn or remember for a long time, he or she may decide it is time to find out why.

Adults should seek qualified professionals to conduct the assessment. These professionals are licensed to evaluate LD and include psychologists and psychiatrists.

The diagnostic process for identifying LDs in adults is similar to that of diagnosing a student.

It includes interviews and observations, testing, an assessment of the results, and recommendations for living with the LD.

The assessment may include:

- **An interview** to gather information about the person's academic and career history, a review of any medical issues, and other information that can help the evaluator with the diagnosis.

- **A career interest inventory** to aid in determining what career areas are matches for the person's interests.

- **Standardized tests** that are selected by the professional based on the information given to them. As with students, these tests can test general ability or specific skills. Standardized tests are used to look at the person's intelligence, achievement, and ability to process information. Based on those results, further tests may be administered to identify specific LDs.

After the professional has gathered enough information, he or she will give the person the results of the assessment including the LD(s) identified and make recommendations for learning and living.

Because each person is different, the diagnosing of learning disabilities must be individually tailored to that person. Age and development play a part in determining whether a person has one or more LDs and which ones they are. In addition, LDs may not appear until later because the person has learned to cope with the LD or it has been masked by other strengths. Regardless of when an LD is first suspected, the final diagnosis must be made by a professional or group of professionals.

References

1. "Adult Learning Disability Assessment Process," Learning Disabilities Association of America, 2016.

2. "Adults with Learning Disabilities—An Overview," Learning Disabilities Association of America, 2016.

3. "How are Learning Disabilities Diagnosed?" National Institutes of Health, *Eunice Kennedy Shriver* National Institute of Child Health and Human Development, February 28, 2014.

4. Griffin, Rayma. "Who Can Diagnose Learning and Attention Issues in Adults?" Understood, 2016.

5. Morin, Amanda. "Understanding the Full Evaluation Process," Understood, July 11, 2014.

6. Patino, Erica. "Types of Behavior Assessments," Understood, May 30, 2014.

7. Patino, Erica. "Types of Intelligence and Achievement Tests," Understood, June 5, 2014.

8. Patino, Erica. "Types of Tests for Language, Motor and Processing Skills," Understood, June 5, 2014.

9. Patino, Erica. "Types of Tests for Reading, Writing and Math," Understood, November 18, 2014.

Chapter 6
Statistics On Learning Disabilities

Percentage Of Child Ages 5 To 17 Years Reported To Have Attention Deficit Hyperactivity Disorder (ADHD)

- From 1997 to 2013, the proportion of children ages 5 to 17 years reported to have ever been diagnosed with ADHD increased from 6.3 percent in 1993 to 10.7 percent in 2012 and 9.9 percent in 2013.

- For the years 2010–2013, the percentage of boys reported to have ADHD (13.7%) was higher than the rate for girls (6%). This difference was statistically significant.In 2010–2013, 11.9 percent of White non-Hispanic children, 10.1 percent of Black non-Hispanic children, 6.2 percent of Hispanic children, 2.1 percent of Asian non-Hispanic children, and 11.8 percent of children of all other races were reported to have ADHD.

- In 2010–2013, 13.1 percent of children from families living below the poverty level were reported to have ADHD compared with 9.1 percent of children from families living at or above the poverty level.

Percentage Of Child Ages 5 To 17 Years Reported To Have Learning Disability (LD)

- In 2013, 8.2 percent of children ages 5 to 17 years had ever been diagnosed with a learning disability. There was little change in this percentage between 1997 and 2013.

About This Chapter: This chapter includes text excerpted from "Neurodevelopmental Disorders," U.S. Environmental Protection Agency (EPA), October 2015.

- For the years 2010–2013, the percentage of boys reported to have a learning disability (10.4%) was higher than for girls (6.6%).

- The reported prevalence of learning disability varies by race and ethnicity. The highest percentages of learning disability are reported for American Indian or Alaska Native non-Hispanic children (12.7%), Black non-Hispanic children (9.8%), children of "All Other Races" (9.6%), and White non-Hispanic children (8.9%). By comparison, 7.6 percent of Hispanic children are reported to have a learning disability, and Asian non-Hispanic children have the lowest prevalence of learning disability, at 3%.

- For the years 2010–2013, the percentage of children reported to have a learning disability was higher for children living below the poverty level (12.8%) compared with those living at or above the poverty level (7.4%).

Percentage Of Child Ages 5 To 17 Years Reported To Have Autism

- The percentage of children ages 5 to 17 years reported to have ever been diagnosed with autism rose from 0.1 percent in 1997 to 1.2 percent in 2013.

- For the years 2010–2013, the rate of reported autism was more than four times higher in boys than in girls, 1.9 percent and 0.4 percent, respectively.

- The reported prevalence of autism varies by race/ethnicity. The highest prevalence of autism is for children of "All Other Races" (1.7%) and White non-Hispanic children (1.4%). Autism prevalence was lower among Asian non-Hispanic children (1.1%), Black non-Hispanic children (0.8%), and Hispanic children (0.9%).

- For the years 2010–2013, the prevalence of autism was similar for children living below the poverty level and those living at or above the poverty level.

In 2013–14, the number of children and youth ages 3–21 receiving special education services was 6.5 million, or about 13 percent of all public school students. Among students receiving special education services, 35 percent had specific learning disabilities.

(Source: "Children And Youth With Disabilities," U.S. Department of Education (ED).)

Part Two
Types Of Learning Disabilities

Chapter 7
Three Categories Of Learning Disabilities

A learning disability (LD) is a neurobiological condition that affects the way individuals of average to above average intelligence:

- receive information
- process information
- express information

LD can affect one or more stages of information processing that are used in learning which include:

- input—the way new information is taken in.
- integration—the way information is organized and understood.
- memory—the way we store information so we can retrieve it again later.
- output—the way we communicate and express information.

When an individual has a LD that affects part or parts of this process it has the potential to negatively impact their ability to acquire basic skills of:

- listening
- speaking
- thinking

About This Chapter: This chapter includes text excerpted from "What Is A Learning Disability?" U.S. Department of Labor (DOL), n.d. Reviewed December 2016.

- reading

- spelling

- writing

- mathematics

Individuals do not have learning disabilities if their learning problems are due primarily to:

- economic disadvantage
- emotional disorders
- lack of educational opportunities due to:
  - English as a second language
  - frequent changes of schools
  - lack of instruction in basic skills
  - poor school attendance
  - normal process of learning a second language
  - physical disabilities

What Are The Types Of Learning Disabilities?

The criteria and characteristics for diagnosing LD appear in the Diagnostic and Statistical Manual of Mental Disorders (DSM-IV). Learning disabilities can be divided into three broad categories:

- **Developmental Speech and Language Disorders**—Individuals with developmental speech and language disorders have difficulty producing speech sounds, using spoken language to communicate, or understanding what other people say.

- **Academic Skills Disorders**—Students with academic skills disorders are often years behind their peers in developing reading, writing, or math skills.

- **Other Learning Disabilities** (a catch-all that includes certain coordination disorders and LD not covered by the other terms)—These diagnoses include delays in acquiring language, academic, and motor skills that can affect the ability to learn, but do not meet the criteria for a specific LD. Also included are coordination disorders that can lead to poor penmanship, as well as certain spelling and memory disorders.

Table 7.1. Common Types Of Learning Disabilities

Learning Disability	Area Of Impact	Symptoms
Dyslexia	Oral and written language	• Difficulty with listening, speaking, reading, and writing
		• Sees letters or words reversed
		• Sees letters or words transposed
		• Omits letters or words when reading
Dyscalculia	Math	• Difficulty performing calculations
		• Difficulty with numbers
		• Spatial problems
		• Difficulty placing numbers into vertical columns
Dysgraphia	Writing	• Illegible handwriting
		• Difficulty writing within a defined space
		• Letter reversals
		• Letter transposition
		• Omission of letters or words
		• Poor spelling
Dyspraxia	Body coordination	• Problems with muscle control and coordination
		• Apparent clumsiness
Sensory Processing	Perception	• Problems understanding visual and auditory information
Specific Learning Disability	Oral and/or written language, math, reading, writing, and perception	• Difficulty understanding or using language, whether written or spoken
		• Imperfect ability to listen, think, speak, write, read, spell, or do mathematical calculations

A person can have more than one learning disability. Learning disabilities can last a person's entire life, but they may be alleviated with the right educational supports.

(Source: "Learning Disabilities," Eunice Kennedy Shriver *National Institute of Child Health and Human Development (NICHD).)*

Chapter 8

Dyslexia: Reading Disability

What Is Dyslexia?

Dyslexia is a type of learning disability. A person with a learning disability has trouble processing words or numbers. There are several kinds of learning disabilities; dyslexia is the term used when people have difficulty learning to read, even though they are smart enough and are motivated to learn. The word dyslexia comes from two Greek words: **dys**, which means abnormal or impaired, and **lexis**, which refers to language or words.

Dyslexia is not a disease. It's a condition that you are born with, and it often runs in families. People with dyslexia are not stupid or lazy. Most have average or above-average intelligence, and they work very hard to overcome their learning problems.

What Causes Dyslexia?

Research has shown that dyslexia happens because of the way the brain processes information. Pictures of the brain, taken with modern imaging tools, have shown that when people with dyslexia read, they use different parts of the brain than people without dyslexia. These pictures also show that the brains of people with dyslexia don't work efficiently during reading. So that's why reading seems like such slow, hard work.

Most people think that dyslexia causes people to reverse letters and numbers and see words backwards. But reversals happen as a normal part of development, and are seen in many kids until first or second grade. The main problem in dyslexia is trouble recognizing **phonemes**, which are the basic sounds of speech (the "b" sound in "bat" is a phoneme, for example).

About This Chapter: Text in this chapter is excerpted from "Understanding Dyslexia," © 1995–2016. The Nemours Foundation/KidsHealth®. Reprinted with permission.

Therefore, it's a struggle to make the connection between the sound and the letter symbol for that sound, and to blend sounds into words.

This makes it hard to recognize short, familiar words or to sound out longer words. It takes a lot of time for a person with dyslexia to sound out a word. The meaning of the word is often lost, and reading comprehension is poor. It is not surprising that people with dyslexia have trouble spelling. They may also have trouble expressing themselves in writing and even speaking. Dyslexia is a **language processing disorder**, so it can affect all forms of language, either spoken or written.

Some people have milder forms of dyslexia, so they may have less trouble in these other areas of spoken and written language. Some people work around their dyslexia, but it takes a lot of effort and extra work. Dyslexia isn't something that goes away on its own or that a person outgrows. Fortunately, with proper help, most people with dyslexia learn to read. They often find different ways to learn and use those strategies all their lives.

What's It Like To Have Dyslexia?

If you have dyslexia, you might have trouble reading even simple words you've seen many times. You probably will read slowly and feel that you have to work extra-hard when reading. You might mix up the letters in a word, for example, reading the word "now" as "won" or "left" as "felt." Words may blend together and spaces are lost. Phrases might appear like this:

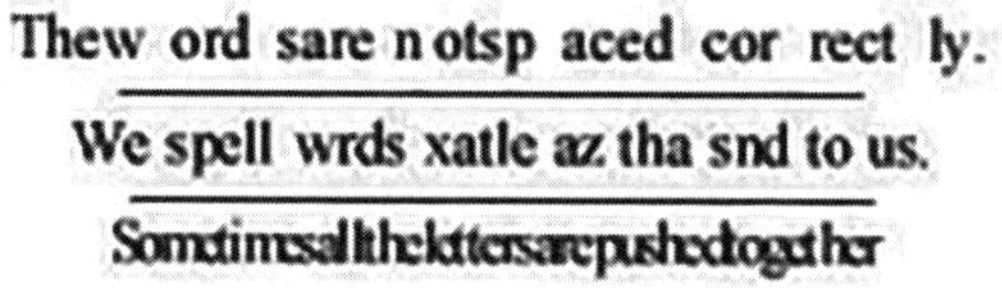

Thew ord sare n otsp aced cor rect ly.

We spell wrds xatle az tha snd to us.

Sometimesallthelettersarepushedtogether

Figure 8.1. Reading Difficulties

You might have trouble remembering what you've read. You may remember more easily when the same information is read to you or heard on tape. Word problems in math may be especially hard, even if you've mastered the basics of arithmetic. If you're doing a presentation in front of the class, you might have trouble finding the right words or names for various objects. Spelling and writing usually are very hard for people with dyslexia.

How Is Dyslexia Diagnosed?

People with dyslexia frequently find ways to work around their disability, so no one will know they're having trouble. This may save some embarrassment, but getting help could make school and reading easier. Most people are diagnosed as kids, but it's not unusual for teens or even adults to be diagnosed.

A teen's parents or teachers might suspect dyslexia if they notice many of these problems:

- poor reading skills, despite having normal intelligence

- poor spelling and writing skills

- difficulty finishing assignments and tests within time limits

- difficulty remembering the right names for things

- difficulty memorizing written lists and phone numbers

- difficulty with directions (telling right from left or up from down) or reading maps

- difficulty getting through foreign language classes

If someone has one of these problems it doesn't mean he or she has dyslexia, but someone who shows several of these signs should be tested for the condition.

A physical exam should be done to rule out any medical problems, including hearing and vision tests. Then a school psychologist or learning specialist should give several standardized tests to measure language, reading, spelling, and writing abilities. Sometimes a test of thinking ability (IQ test) is given. Some people with dyslexia have trouble in other school skills, like handwriting and math, or they may have trouble paying attention or remembering things. If this is the case, more testing will be done.

Dealing With Dyslexia

Although dealing with dyslexia can be tough, help is available. Under federal law, some-one diagnosed with a learning disability like dyslexia is entitled to extra help from the public school system. A child or teen with dyslexia usually needs to work with a specially trained teacher, tutor, or reading specialist to learn how to read and spell better. The best type of help teaches awareness of speech sounds in words (called **phonemic awareness**) and letter-sound correspondences (called **phonics**). The teacher or tutor should use special learning and practice activities for dyslexia.

A student with dyslexia may get more time to complete assignments or tests, permission to tape class lectures, or copies of lecture notes. Using a computer with spelling checkers can be helpful for written assignments. For older students in challenging classes, services are available that provide any book on tape, even textbooks. Computer software is also available that "reads" printed material aloud. Ask your parent, teacher, or learning disability services coordinator how to get these services if you need them.

Treatment with eye exercises or glasses with tinted lenses will not help a person with dyslexia. It's not an eye problem, it's a language processing problem, so teaching language processing skills is the most important part of treatment.

Emotional support for people with dyslexia is very important. They often get frustrated because no matter how hard they try, they can't seem to keep up with other students. They often feel that they are stupid or worthless, and may cover up their difficulties by acting up in class or by becoming the class clown. They may try to get other students to do their work for them. They may pretend that they don't care about their grades or that they think school is dumb.

Family and friends can help people with dyslexia by understanding that they aren't stupid or lazy, and that they are trying as hard as they can. It's important to recognize and appreciate each person's strengths, whether they're in sports, drama, art, creative problem solving, or something else.

People with dyslexia shouldn't feel limited in their academic or career choices. Most colleges make special accommodations for students with dyslexia, offering them trained tutors, learning aids, computer software, reading assignments on tape, and special arrangements for exams. People with dyslexia can become doctors, politicians, corporate executives, actors, musicians, artists, teachers, inventors, business entrepreneurs, or whatever else they choose.

Chapter 9
Dysgraphia: Writing Disability

You probably hear a lot about learning and attention issues like dyslexia and Attention-deficit hyperactivity disorder (ADHD). But chances are you don't hear much about dysgraphia. If your child has trouble expressing himself in writing, you may want to learn more about this condition.

Writing difficulties are common among children and can stem from a variety of learning and attention issues. By learning what to watch for, you can be proactive about getting help for your child.

There's no cure or easy fix for dysgraphia. But there are strategies and therapies that can help a child improve his writing. This will help him thrive in school and anywhere else expressing himself in writing is important.

What Is Dysgraphia?

Dysgraphia is a condition that causes trouble with written expression. The term comes from the Greek words dys ("impaired") and graphia ("making letter forms by hand"). Dysgraphia is a brain-based issue. It's not the result of a child being lazy.

For many children with dysgraphia, just holding a pencil and organizing letters on a line is difficult. Their handwriting tends to be messy. Many struggle with spelling and putting thoughts on paper. These and other writing tasks—like putting ideas into language that is organized, stored and then retrieved from memory—may all add to struggles with written expression.

About This Chapter: Text in this chapter is excerpted from "Understanding Dysgraphia," © 2014–2016 Understood.org USA LLC. Reprinted with permission.

Different professionals may use different terms to describe your child's struggle with written expression. The Diagnostic and Statistical Manual of Mental Disorders-5 (DSM-5) doesn't use the term dysgraphia but uses the phrase "an impairment in written expression" under the category of "specific learning disorder." This is the term used by most doctors and psychologists.

Some school psychologists and teachers use the term dysgraphia as a type of shorthand to mean "a disorder in written expression."

To qualify for special education services, a child must have an issue named or described in the Individuals with Disabilities Education Act (IDEA). While IDEA doesn't use the term "dysgraphia," it describes it under the category of "specific learning disability." This includes issues with understanding or using language (spoken or written) that make it difficult to listen, think, speak, read, write, spell or to do mathematical calculations.

Whatever definition is used, it's important to understand that slow or sloppy writing isn't necessarily a sign that your child isn't trying hard enough. Writing requires a complex set of fine motor and language processing skills. For kids with dysgraphia, the writing process is harder and slower. Without help, a child with dysgraphia may have a difficult time in school.

How Common Is Dysgraphia?

Dysgraphia is not a familiar term. But symptoms of dysgraphia are not uncommon, especially in young children who are starting to learn how to write. If a child continues to struggle with writing despite plenty of practice and corrective feedback, it's a good idea to take a closer look to see whether dysgraphia is an underlying cause.

What Causes Dysgraphia?

Experts aren't sure what causes dysgraphia and other issues of written expression. Normally, the brain takes in information through the senses and stores it to use later. Before a person starts writing, he retrieves information from his short- or long-term memory and gets organized to begin writing.

In a person with dysgraphia, experts believe one or both of the next steps in the writing process go off track:

1. Organizing information that is stored in memory

2. Getting words onto paper by handwriting or typing them

This results in a written product that's hard to read and filled with errors. And most important, it does not convey what the child knows and what he intended to write.

Working memory may also play a role in dysgraphia. A child may have trouble with what's called "**orthographic coding**." This is the ability to store unfamiliar written words in the working memory. As a result, he may have a hard time remembering how to print or write a letter or a word.

There may also be a genetic link, with dysgraphia running in families.

What Are The Symptoms Of Dysgraphia?

The symptoms of dysgraphia fall into six categories: visual-spatial, fine motor, language processing, spelling/handwriting, grammar, and organization of language. A child may have dysgraphia if his writing skills lag behind those of his peers and he has at least some of these symptoms:

Visual-Spatial Difficulties

- Has trouble with shape-discrimination and letter spacing
- Has trouble organizing words on the page from left to right
- Writes letters that go in all directions, and letters and words that run together on the page
- Has a hard time writing on a line and inside margins
- Has trouble reading maps, drawing or reproducing a shape
- Copies text slowly

Fine Motor Difficulties

- Has trouble holding a pencil correctly, tracing, cutting food, tying shoes, doing puzzles, texting and keyboarding
- Is unable to use scissors well or to color inside the lines
- Holds his wrist, arm, body or paper in an awkward position when writing

Language Processing Issues

- Has trouble getting ideas down on paper quickly
- Has trouble understanding the rules of games
- Has a hard time following directions
- Loses his train of thought

Spelling/Handwriting Issues

- Has a hard time understanding spelling rules
- Has trouble telling if a word is misspelled
- Can spell correctly orally but makes spelling errors in writing
- Spells words incorrectly and in many different ways
- Has trouble using spell-check—and when he does, he doesn't recognize the correct word
- Mixes upper- and lowercase letters
- Blends printing and cursive
- Has trouble reading his own writing
- Avoids writing
- Gets a tired or cramped handed when he writes
- Erases a lot

Grammar and Usage Problems

- Doesn't know how to use punctuation
- Overuses commas and mixes up verb tenses
- Doesn't start sentences with a capital letter
- Doesn't write in complete sentences but writes in a list format
- Writes sentences that "run on forever"

Organization of Written Language

- Has trouble telling a story and may start in the middle
- Leaves out important facts and details, or provides too much information
- Assumes others know what he's talking about
- Uses vague descriptions
- Writes jumbled sentences
- Never gets to the point, or makes the same point over and over
- Is better at conveying ideas when speaking

The symptoms of dysgraphia also vary depending on a child's age. Signs generally appear when children are first learning to write.

- **Preschool children** may be hesitant to write and draw and say that they hate coloring.

- **School-age children** may have illegible handwriting that can be mix of cursive and print. They may have trouble writing on a line and may print letters that are uneven in size and height. Some children also may need to say words out loud when writing or have trouble putting their thoughts on paper.

- **Teenagers** may write in simple sentences. Their writing may have many more grammatical mistakes than the writing of other kids their age.

What Skills Are Affected By Dysgraphia?

The impact of dysgraphia on a child's development varies, depending on the symptoms and their severity. Here are some common areas of struggle for kids with dysgraphia:

- **Academic:** Kids with dysgraphia can fall behind in schoolwork because it takes them so much longer to write. Taking notes is a challenge. They may get discouraged and avoid writing assignments.

- **Basic life skills:** Some children's fine motor skills are weak. They find it hard to do everyday tasks, such as buttoning shirts and making a simple list.

- **Social-emotional:** Children with dysgraphia may feel frustrated or anxious about their academic and life challenges. If they haven't been identified, teachers may criticize them for being "lazy" or "sloppy." This may add to their stress. Their low self-esteem, frustration and communication problems can also make it hard to socialize with other children.

While dysgraphia is a lifelong condition, there are many proven strategies and tools that can help children with dysgraphia improve their writing skills.

How Is Dysgraphia Diagnosed?

Signs of dysgraphia often appear in early elementary school. But the signs may not become apparent until middle school or later. Sometimes the signs go unnoticed entirely. As with all learning and attention issues, the earlier signs of dysgraphia are recognized and addressed, the better.

Dysgraphia is typically identified by licensed psychologists (including school psychologists) who specialize in learning disabilities. They will give your child academic assessments and writing tests. These tests measure fine motor skills and written expression production.

During testing, the professional may ask your child to write sentences and copy text. They'll assess not only your child's finished product, but also his writing process. This includes posture, position, pencil grip, fatigue and whether there are signs of cramping. The tester may also test fine motor speed with finger tapping and wrist turning.

Special education teachers and school psychologists can help determine the emotional or academic impact the condition may be having on your child.

What Conditions Are Related To Dysgraphia?

Many children with dysgraphia have other learning issues. These conditions, which can also affect written expression, include:

- **Dyslexia:** This learning issue makes it harder to read. Dyslexia can also make writing and spelling a challenge.

- **Language disorders:** Language disorders can cause a variety of problems with written and spoken language. Children may have trouble learning new words, using correct grammar and putting their thoughts into words.

- **Attention-deficit hyperactivity disorder (ADHD):** ADHD causes problems with attention, impulsivity and hyperactivity.

- **Dyspraxia:** Dyspraxia is a condition that causes poor physical coordination and motor skills. It can cause trouble with fine motor skills, which can affect physical task of writing and printing.

How Can Professionals Help With Dysgraphia?

If your child is found to have dysgraphia and qualifies for special education services, you and a team of teachers and specialists at the school will develop an Individualized Education Program (IEP). This may include intensive instruction in handwriting as well as personalized accommodations and modifications.

If your child isn't eligible for an IEP, another option is to request a 504 plan. This is a written plan that details how the school will accommodate your child's needs.

But even without an IEP or 504 plan, you may be able to get help in other ways:

- Response to intervention (RTI) is an approach some schools use to screen students and provide small group instruction to those who are falling behind. If a child doesn't make progress, he may receive intensive one-on-one instruction.

- Informal supports are strategies your child's teacher can use, such as giving your child copies of class notes or using assistive technology tools like voice-to-text (dictation) software.

There are many ways to help a child with dysgraphia. Generally, support falls into these categories:

- **Accommodations** are changes to how your child learns. Accommodations include typing on a keyboard or other electronic device instead of writing by hand. Apps can help some children stay organized through voice-recorded notes.

- **Modifications** are changes to what your child learns. Examples of modifications include allowing a student to write shorter papers or answer fewer or different test questions than his classmates.

- **Remediation** is an approach that targets foundational skills your child needs to master. Some children may practice copying letters, using paper with raised lines to help them write in straight lines. An occupational therapist may provide exercises to build muscle strength and dexterity and increase hand-eye coordination.

There is no medication for treating dysgraphia. However, children who also have ADHD sometimes find that medication for ADHD alleviates symptoms of dysgraphia.

What Can Be Done At Home For Dysgraphia?

There are many things you can do at home to help your child with dysgraphia. Here are some strategies to consider.

- **Observe and take notes.** Taking notes about your child's writing difficulties (including when they occur) will help you find patterns and triggers. Then you can develop strategies to work around them. Your notes will also be useful when you talk to your child's doctor, teachers and anyone else helping your child.

- **Teach your child writing warm-up exercises.** Before writing (or even as a break when writing), your child can do a stress-reliever exercise. He could shake his hands quickly or rub them together to relieve tension.

- **Play games that strengthen motor skills.** Playing with clay can strengthen hand muscles. A squeeze ball can improve hand and wrist muscles and coordination.

It's best not to try too many strategies at once. Instead, add one at a time so you know what is (or isn't) working. Praise your child for effort and genuine achievement. This can motivate him to keep building skills. Many kids overcome and work around their writing difficulties. With support, your child can, too.

Chapter 10

Dyscalculia: Math Disability

What Is Dyscalculia?

Dyscalculia is not as well known as dyslexia, but both are learning disabilities.

Dyscalculia = Math

Causes trouble with

- understanding arithmetic (numbers) concepts and solving arithmetic problems

- estimating time, measuring, and budgeting

Also called a **Math Learning Disability.**

Dyslexia = Written language

Causes trouble with

- spelling
- understanding written sentences
- recognizing printed words seen before

Also called a **Reading Disability.**

About This Chapter: Text beginning with the heading "What Is Dyscalculia?" is excerpted from "Does Your Child Struggle With Math?" *Eunice Kennedy Shriver* National Institute of Child Health and Human Development (NICHD), April 22, 2016; Text beginning with the heading "Symptoms," is © 2017 Omnigraphics. Reviewed January 2017.

How Many People Have Dyscalculia?

- More than 20 million people.

- Boys are slightly more likely to have dyscalculia than girls.

What Are The Risk Factors For Dyscalculia?

By age 4

Has trouble

- listing numbers in correct order

- matching number words or written digits to number of objects

- counting objects

Age 6–12

Has regular and lasting trouble

- performing addition, subtraction, multiplication, or division appropriate to grade level

- recognizing math errors

Age 12+

Has trouble

- estimating (informed guessing)

- making exact calculations

- understanding graphs and charts

- understanding fractions and decimals

How Can Adults Reduce The Risk Of Dyscalculia In Young Children?

Show the child that numbers are a normal part of everyday life.

- Mention numbers to your child while doing everyday activities—like grocery shopping or setting the table.

- Count out loud and show the child both the written number word ("three") and digit ("3").

- Count actual objects the child can see.

- Compare objects in everyday conversation using words that describe size or amount.

Symptoms

In early childhood, dyscalculia is typified by general difficulty with numbers, recognizing patterns, and sorting objects by shape or size. As children enter school and math learning progresses, the characteristics may include trouble with simple addition, subtraction, multiplication, and division, as well as difficulty retaining numerical concepts and applying math to common situations.

Teens with dyscalculia continue to have problems as math becomes increasingly complex and more is expected of them. Symptoms for this age group, as well as adults, can include:

- Lack of understanding of time, often late or miscalculating how long tasks will take.

- Difficulty applying math principles to everyday life, such as calculating the area of a room or the amount of a tip.

- Poor sense of direction, easily gets lost or worries about getting lost.

- Trouble judging distances between objects.

- May do well in classes that require reading and writing skills, such as english and history, but struggles in those that rely on numbers, like algebra and science.

- Trouble with measurements, as in recipes or woodworking, especially when conversions are necessary (pints to ounces, for example).

- Difficulty understanding information in chart or graph form.

- Good recall of spoken or printed words, but has trouble remembering numbers and patterns.

> It's not unusual for dyscalculia to co-occur with other types of learning difficulties, such as attention deficit hyperactivity disorder (ADHD), dyslexia, or dyspraxia (problems with movement), so evaluation will often include testing for these conditions, as well.

Diagnosis

Most often, various types of learning disabilities are identified when children are quite young, and this is usually the case with dyscalculia. But often younger students do so well in other areas, and the level of math being taught is simple enough, that they are able to mask the symptoms. As a result, in some cases dyscalculia may not be diagnosed until the teen years, when work with numbers becomes considerably more complex and students start to fall behind.

There is no single cause for dyscalculia, but because some of the underlying problems can be neurological or genetic, the first step in diagnosis should be a physical examination by a doctor who is aware that the teen has been exhibiting some of the above symptoms. If no physical cause can be determined, then the student should be evaluated by a specialist in learning disabilities, who will review past performance, administer a variety of tests, and ask questions to determine the individual's skills and understanding of various concepts. Some of the evaluation process will likely include:

- Questions about areas in which the teen feels he or she has had difficulty.

- Questions about times when the student has felt hopeless or frustrated about math.

- Probing for other learning disabilities that may be contributing factors

- An evaluation of basic math skills (counting, addition, subtraction, etc.).

- Determining whether the teen can discern patterns and organize objects logically.

- Testing for the ability to estimate quantity.

- Gauging the individual's facility with money (making change, estimating costs, etc.).

- Evaluating the ability to tell time and determine how long tasks will take.

- Assessing the student's ability to find alternate ways to solve problems.

An important part of diagnosis is to evaluate how well the teen is able to understand math concepts and apply them to common situations, rather than just having him or her perform a series of calculations. For math learning to move forward, it's critical that the student develop a solid grasp of underlying principles, and this won't happen without an accurate assessment of his or her history and current status.

Students who have been diagnosed with dyscalculia may be eligible for special classroom accommodation or other support under the Individuals with Disabilities Education Act (IDEA). Ask a school guidance counselor, special education teacher, or the principal's office for more information.

(Source: "Dyslexia Guidance," U.S. Department of Education (ED).)

Treatment

Dyscalculia cannot be cured, and it won't improve on its own. But with treatment by a trained professional, along with dedication on the part of the student and support from teachers, parents, and peers, math skills can be improved considerably. Some strategies include:

- Helping students be aware of their strengths and weaknesses so they can understand and make use of their own unique learning style.

- Devising real-life examples that link math skills to everyday situations.

- Breaking complex problems into smaller, more easily managed parts.

- Using visual aids, such as drawings or physical objects, to help solve math problems.

- Talking through the problem-solving process verbally.

- Using graph paper to help organize ideas.

- Working on a calculator when this is appropriate.

- Circling computation signs before trying to solve a problem.

- Covering up most of a math exercise or test with a piece of paper to make it easier to concentrate on one problem at a time.

- Playing math-related video games.

- Reading math problems aloud and continuing to talk while working on a solution.

- Reviewing new skills, discussing, and asking questions before moving on to the next task.

- Engaging a tutor to help with review, practice, and any particular areas of difficulty.

- Working with a classmate or other peer on homework assignments or to review the day's lessons.

References

1. "Dyscalculia," National Center for Learning Disabilities, 2007.

2. "Dyscalculia: Indications, Treatment and Strategies," NoBullying.com, September 4, 2016.

3. Morin, Amanda. "Treatment Options for Dyscalculia," Understood.org, n.d.

4. Morin, Amanda. "Understanding Dyscalculia," Understood.org, n.d.

5. "What is Dyscalculia?" Dyslexia SPELD Foundation, 2014.

Chapter 11
Developmental Speech And Language Disorders

It's not unusual for very young children to have difficulty understanding and expressing themselves, but some people continue to experience language problems, often into adolescence and adulthood. Teens with speech and language disorders may have trouble communicating with their peers, teachers, parents, and other adults. As they get older and classroom work requires more advanced oral and written communication skills, their school work may suffer. Beyond that, language disorders in teens can lead to low self-esteem, poor interpersonal relationships, and difficulty in the workforce. When these issues are addressed early through professional intervention, the majority of children show considerable improvement, but for some individuals treatment will continue as they get older, and for those who never received professional attention at a young age, evaluation and treatment may begin during the teen or adult years.

> Speech and language disorders are among the most common disabilities facing children and adolescents. According to government statistics, such disorders affect approximately 4.9 percent of U.S. students aged 11 to 17, in addition to even larger numbers of younger children.
>
> *(Source: "Quick Statistics About Voice, Speech, Language," National Institute on Deafness and Other Communication Disorders (NIDCD).)*

Speech Disorders

A speech disorder is a condition that occurs when a person has difficulty producing the sounds needed to communicate effectively with others. These are often divided into four major types:

"Developmental Speech And Language Disorders," © 2017 Omnigraphics. Reviewed January 2017.

- **Articulation.** Articulation refers to the way people make sounds, and those with an articulation disorder may distort, substitute, or leave out some of the sounds used to produce "normal" speech. For example, they may substitute a "w" for an "r" ("wobin" for "robin") or leave out a portion of a word ("nana" instead of "banana").

- **Phonology.** Phonological disorders are very closely related to articulation (in fact, many experts classify them together), but phonology refers to the way speech sounds are organized and the way the brain works to sort them out. As children learn to speak, they tend to simplify language in their minds, substituting easier letters for more difficult ones, or just eliminating portions of words to make them easier to say. When individuals don't move beyond this simplification, it is considered a disorder.

- **Voice.** Sometimes called vocal disorders, these are characterized by the inability to produce a clear sound and can include difficulty with volume, pitch, or other qualities associated with clear communication. Examples include hoarseness, extremely loud speech, very high or low pitch, nasal speech, or occasional total loss of voice.

- **Fluency.** A fluency disorder is one that interferes with the smoothness, continuity, and normal rate of speech. It can include the repetition of sounds or entire words, broken words, gaps in speech, and prolongation of certain sounds. The most common fluency problem is stuttering, which typically begins in childhood and, in some cases, may last a lifetime, to a greater or lesser degree.

Language Disorders

A person with a language disorder has difficulty understanding what is being said by others, finding the right words to communicate clearly, or both. There are three primary types of language disorders:

- **Receptive language disorders.** Individuals with receptive language disorders have problems understanding, retaining, and processing spoken language. Although symptoms vary considerably, they can include appearing not to listen, inability to comprehend complex sentences, difficulty following conversations, and inability to follow instructions.

- **Expressive language disorders.** Those with expressive language disorders have difficulty putting words and sentences together, verbally or in writing, in a cohesive and appropriate manner. The condition is characterized by limited vocabulary, difficulty recalling words, poor grammar, and the inability to put sentences together to tell a coherent story.

- **Mixed language disorders.** A mixed receptive-expressive language disorder is one in which an individual has trouble both understanding others and expressing him- or herself effectively. The outward characteristics of this condition are essentially the same as those of expressive language disorder but may also include inappropriate responses to communication or the inability to follow instructions.

Diagnosis

Sometimes speech and language disorders are caused by such conditions as hearing loss, brain injury, neurological problems, or physical issues in the mouth or throat, and in these cases a physician will most likely form a diagnosis. But more often the cause of the disorder is unknown, making diagnosis by a trained specialist necessary.

There are a number of standardized tests specifically aimed at children from birth to six years of age that are routinely administered to arrive at a diagnosis and help develop a treatment plan. Even though there has been less attention paid to the formal evaluation of speech and language issues in teens, there are some standardized tests that, combined with general observation, interviews, and a review of classroom performance, can be useful in obtaining a diagnosis. Some of these include:

- **Peabody Picture Test.** Designed in 1959 and updated several times since then, this test is administered to children, teens, and adults to determine receptive vocabulary ability. During the test, the examiner shows the individual being evaluated a series of pictures then says a word and has the subject identify the picture that best illustrates the word. Results are then compared to standardized norms for the age group.

- **The Listening Comprehension Test Adolescent.** Intended for individuals aged 12 to 17, this test evaluates the student's ability to listen and comprehend language that would typically be used in a classroom setting. During testing, the subject listens to a story and then answers questions posed by the examiner, some of which relate to understanding of the story's meaning, some to vocabulary, and others to recall of information.

- **The Word Test 2 Adolescent.** This test measures an individual's ability to understand the meaning of words, using six skill areas to evaluate both classroom and common language usage. These include identifying a synonym for a given word, providing an antonym for a given word, choosing the unrelated word among four, defining words, repairing an absurd statement, and giving multiple meanings for words.

- **Social Language Development Test Adolescent.** This evaluation assesses such areas as the teen's ability to interpret social language, engage in social interactions, take on someone else's perspective, and devise solutions to social problems based on language used in the interaction. The procedure involves a variety of pictures, stories, and role-playing exercises.

There are many other tests that professionals who specialize in working with teens may use to help diagnose speech and language problems, including those that evaluate spelling, writing, reading comprehension, memory, and vocabulary.

Treatment

Because of the complexity and numerous types of speech and language disorders, treatment plans vary considerably from case to case. Ideally, the cooperation of specialized professionals, parents, school systems, teachers, and peers will help ensure the best possible outcome:

- Speech therapists and language specialists can work individually with the student to help improve pronunciation, vocabulary, and grammar skills.

- Psychologists may be engaged if the student has emotional issues related to, or underlying, speech or language disorders.

- Public schools are required under the Individuals with Disabilities Education Act (IDEA) to provide special educational programs for qualified individuals, so those with language disorders might be able to get help through the school system.

- Although teachers may not be specially trained in speech therapy, after discussions with parents and professionals, they will likely be able to make accommodations for students who have language difficulty. For example, they might allow alternative means of communication for some students, or they could modify homework assignments to meet those students' needs.

- Peers can be a great source of practice or reinforcement. Those who have speech or language disorders themselves can form part of a network to work with each other on various exercises. And peers who do not have such disorders can be enlisted to serve as role models and sources of feedback for their friends or classmates who need extra help in this area.

Public schools can help teens with speech and language disorders in a number of ways. Qualified students can work with their parents, educators, and professionals to develop an Individualized Education Program (IEP), which could include classroom assistance, homework plans, and speech therapy.

References

1. Clark, Mary Kristen, MS, and Alan G. Kamhi, Ph.D. "Language Disorders," International Encyclopedia of Rehabilitation, 2010.

2. Elleseff, Tatyana, MA, CCC-SLP. "Comprehensive Assessment of Adolescents with Suspected Language and Literacy Disorders," SmartSpeechTherapy.com, October 9, 2016.

3. "Speech and Language Disorders," Bright Minds Institute, n.d.

4. "Speech and Language Impairments," Center for Parent Information and Resources, January 2011.

5. "Speech and Language Therapy," Kaufman Children's Center, 2016.

6. "Understanding Language Disorders," Understood.org, n.d.

Chapter 12

Specific Language Impairment (SLI)

What Is Specific Language Impairment?

Specific language impairment (SLI) is a language disorder that delays the mastery of language skills in children who have no hearing loss or other developmental delays. SLI is also called developmental language disorder, language delay, or developmental dysphasia. It is one of the most common childhood learning disabilities, affecting approximately 7 to 8 percent of children in kindergarten. The impact of SLI persists into adulthood.

What Causes Specific Language Impairment?

The cause of SLI is unknown, but recent discoveries suggest it has a strong genetic link. Children with SLI are more likely than those without SLI to have parents and siblings who also have had difficulties and delays in speaking. In fact, 50 to 70 percent of children with SLI have at least one other family member with the disorder.

What Are The Symptoms Of Specific Language Impairment?

Children with SLI are often late to talk and may not produce any words until they are 2 years old. At age 3, they may talk, but may not be understood. As they grow older, children with SLI will struggle to learn new words and make conversation. Having difficulty using verbs is a hallmark of SLI. Typical errors that a 5-year-old child with SLI would make include dropping the "s" from the end of present-tense verbs, dropping past tense, and asking questions without the usual

About This Chapter: This chapter includes text excerpted from "Specific Language Impairment," National Institute on Deafness and Other Communication Disorders (NIDCD), April 24, 2015.

"be" or "do" verbs. For example, instead of saying "She rides the horse," a child with SLI will say, "She ride the horse." Instead of saying "He ate the cookie," a child with SLI will say, "He eat the cookie." Instead of saying "Why does he like me?", a child with SLI will ask, "Why he like me?".

What Is The Difference Between A Speech Disorder And A Language Disorder?

Children who have trouble understanding what others say (receptive language) or difficulty sharing their thoughts (expressive language) may have a language disorder. Specific language impairment (SLI) is a language disorder that delays the mastery of language skills. Some children with SLI may not begin to talk until their third or fourth year.

Children who have trouble producing speech sounds correctly or who hesitate or stutter when talking may have a speech disorder. Apraxia of speech is a speech disorder that makes it difficult to put sounds and syllables together in the correct order to form words.

(Source: "Speech And Language Developmental Milestones," National Institute on Deafness and Other Communication Disorders (NIDCD).)

How Is Specific Language Impairment Diagnosed In Children?

The first person to suspect a child might have SLI is often a parent or preschool or school teacher. A number of speech-language professionals might be involved in the diagnosis, including a speech-language pathologist (a health professional trained to evaluate and treat children with speech or language problems). Language skills are tested using assessment tools that evaluate how well the child constructs sentences and keeps words in their proper order, the number of words in his or her vocabulary, and the quality of his or her spoken language. There are a number of tests commercially available that can specifically diagnose SLI. Some of the tests use interactions between the child and puppets and other toys to focus on specific rules of grammar, especially the misuse of verb tenses. These tests can be used with children between 3 and 8 years of age and are especially useful for identifying children with SLI once they enter school.

What Treatments Are Available For Specific Language Impairment?

Because SLI affects reading it also affects learning. If it is not treated early, it can affect a child's performance in school. Since the early signs of SLI are often present in children as young as 3 years old, the preschool years can be used to prepare them for kindergarten with special programs designed to enrich language development. This kind of classroom program might enlist normally developing children to act as role models for children with SLI and feature activities that encourage role-playing and sharing time, as well as hands-on lessons to explore new, interesting vocabulary. Some parents also might want their child to see a speech-language pathologist, who can assess their child's needs, engage him or her in structured activities, and recommend home materials for at-home enrichment.

What Kinds Of Research Are Being Conducted?

The National Institute on Deafness and Other Communication Disorders (NIDCD) supports a wide variety of research to understand the genetic underpinnings of SLI, the nature of the language deficits that cause it, and better ways to diagnose and treat children with it.

- **Genetic research:** An NIDCD-supported investigator recently has identified a mutation in a gene on chromosome 6, called the *KIAA0319* gene, that appears to play a key role in SLI. The mutation plays a supporting role in other learning disabilities, such as dyslexia, some cases of autism, and speech sound disorders (conditions in which speech sounds are either not produced or produced or used incorrectly). This finding lends support to the idea that difficulties in learning language may be coming from the same genes that influence difficulties with reading and understanding printed text. Other potentially influential genes also are being explored.

- **Bilingual research:** The standardized tests that speech-language pathologists use in schools to screen for language impairments are based on typical language development milestones in English. Because bilingual children are more likely to score in the at-risk range on these tests, it becomes difficult to distinguish between children who are struggling to learn a new language and children with true language impairments. After studying a large group of Hispanic children who speak English as a second language, NIDCD-funded researchers have developed a dual language diagnostic test to identify bilingual children with language impairments. It's now being tested in a group of children 4 to 6 years old, and will eventually be expanded to children 7 to 9 years old. The same research team is also trying out an intervention program with a small group of bilingual first graders with SLI to find techniques and strategies to help them succeed academically.

- **Diagnostic research:** Children with SLI have significant communication problems, which are also characteristic of most children with autism spectrum disorders (ASD). Impairments in understanding and the onset of spoken language are common in both groups. No one knows yet if there are early developmental signs that could signal or predict language difficulties and might potentially allow for early identification and intervention with these children. The NIDCD is currently funding researchers looking for risk markers associated with SLI and ASD that could signal later problems in speech and communication. In a group of children 6 months to 1-year old who, because of family history, are at risk for SLI or ASD, the investigators are collecting data using behavioral, eye-tracking, and neurophysiological measures, as well as general measures of cognitive and brain development. They will then follow these children until they are 3 years old to see if there are indicators that are specific to SLI or ASD or that could predict the development of either disorder. Findings from this research could have a major influence in developing new approaches to early screening and diagnosis for SLI and ASD.

Chapter 13
Nonverbal Learning Disability (NLD)

Nonverbal learning disability (NLD) is a brain-based learning disability where individuals have difficulty with abstract thinking, spatial relationships, and identifying and interpreting concepts and patterns. Nonverbal learning disability occurs in 0.1 to 1 percent of the general population. It is also called nonverbal learning disorder (NVLD) or a right-hemisphere learning disorder.

People use the spoken word in various ways. Sometimes they say exactly what they mean. Sometimes they expect the listener to pick up another meaning from their facial expression or tone of voice. Sometimes they expect the listener to fill in information from past experience or some other source of information. For example "I love rainy days" when said directly is the truth. But, if the same phrase is said with a frown or eye roll and a growly tone, the speaker is being sarcastic, and is really telling the listener that she hates rainy days. Finally, if the speaker says, "You know how I feel about rainy days," the listener is expected to fill in some previously learned information. A person with a nonverbal learning disability cannot interpret the facial expressions and tone of voice of the sarcasm and thus takes the untrue statement as true. Nor can the listener draw on a pattern of previously learned information, and thus truly does not know how the speaker feels.

Signs Of NLD

Children with NLD tend to be very smart. They talk freely, develop large vocabularies in comparison to other children their age, memorize facts, and read early. Intelligence tests show high verbal IQ (intelligence quotient) but low performance IQ due to visual-spatial difficulties. There are five main areas of weakness in people with NLD. People with NLD may not

"Nonverbal Learning Disability," © 2017 Omnigraphics. Reviewed June 2016.

exhibit weakness in all five areas, nor may they exhibit them all at once. The weaknesses tend to become more obvious as children progress in school and are required to rely more on identifying patterns and less on memorized facts.

The five main areas of weakness have been identified as:

1. **Visual/Spatial Awareness.** Children with NLD may have problems estimating distance, size, and/or shape of objects. They may be clumsy, spill drinks, bump into people or objects, or not be able to catch a ball. They may also have a poor sense of direction, such as being able to distinguish left from right.

2. **Motor Skills.** Children with NLD may have trouble mastering basic motor skills both large (such as dressing themselves, running, or riding a bike) or small (such as writing or using scissors).

3. **Abstract Thinking.** Children with NLD may have difficulty seeing or understanding the big picture. They can read a story and relate the details, but cannot answer questions about how the details fit together.

4. **Conceptual Skills.** Children with NLD may have trouble grasping the larger concept of a situation. For example, determining how pieces of a puzzle fit together to make a whole or identifying the steps needed to solve a problem. This contributes to problems especially with math.

5. **Social Skills.** Children with NLD may have trouble making friends or socializing in a group. They may interrupt or behave inappropriately in social situations. They use previously learned skills to cope with new social situations, whether appropriate or not.

In addition, because NLD occurs in the right side of the brain, children with NLD may have a distorted sense of touch or feel and poor coordination on the left side of the body.

These areas of weakness are often masked in pre-school and the early elementary grades when students are learning basic (rote) skills like reading and arithmetic. By the fourth or fifth grade, when students are required to process what they read or remember patterns from previous examples, the weaknesses start to become evident. At the same time, these very smart children may start exhibiting behavioral problems brought on by frustration in not "getting it" or feelings of being a social reject.

Diagnosis Of NLD

The diagnosis of NLD is controversial. NLD is not listed in the American Psychiatric Association's Diagnostic and Statistical Manual of Mental Disorders, 5th ed. (DSM-5), the manual used by doctors and therapists to diagnose learning disabilities. Nor is NLD recognized as a disability covered by the Individuals with Disabilities Education Act (IDEA). Nonetheless, if a child is exhibiting signs of NLD, there are steps parents should take to identify the problem.

- **A medical exam.** A thorough physical examination and a discussion of the child's learning problems will help the doctor rule out any physical causes for the learning problems.

- **A mental health professional.** Most likely the family doctor will refer the child to a neurologist or other specialist. The specialist will talk to the parents and child about what is happening, and may administer a variety of tests in the areas of speech and language, motor skills, and visual-spatial relationships. The results coupled with information from the parents and child will help the specialist analyze the strengths and weaknesses associated with NLD and make a diagnosis.

As with many learning disorders, the symptoms of NLD vary from child to child, thus a comprehensive assessment is needed to determine the individual child's needs. With the input and support of learning professionals and therapists as well as the family, steps can be taken to help the student with NLD.

Help For NLD

It is important to work with the child's school specialists to develop accommodations for the child's NLD. Formal accommodations may be developed through an Individualized Education Program (IEP) or 504 plan. If the child does not qualify for either plan, informal accommodations may be made in the classroom. Classroom accommodations may include modifying homework assignments and tests for time and content, presenting lectures with PowerPoint slides so the student can see as well as hear the material being covered, and/or working with a reading specialist to read a passage aloud then extract key terms and ideas.

Parents can help their child in various ways that will make things easier for both the student and the family. They can:

- Establish structure and routine

- Give clear instructions

- Keep a chart of the day's activities, both social and academic

- Make transitions easier by giving logical, step-by-step explanations of what is going to happen (We are going to IHOP restaurant for dinner. We need to leave in an hour.)

- Break down tasks into small steps in a logical sequence

- Play games with the child to have her identify emotions from facial expressions or voice tone

- Avoid sarcasm, or if it happens, use the experience to help the child identify the signs of sarcasm

- Set up one-on-one play dates with another child who shares an interest with yours. Play dates should be structured, monitored, and time bound

- Avoid situations that may overwhelm the child with too much sensory input–noise, smell, activity

There are other sources of help for parents and students. Social skills groups help the student in social situations. Parent behavioral training helps parents learn how to collaborate with teachers. Occupational and physical therapy may help the child improve movement and writing skills as well as build tolerance for outside experiences. Cognitive therapy can help the child deal with anxiety, depression, and other mental health issues.

Although NLD presents many challenges for both the student and the family, there is help available and with patience and effort, there will be improvement.

References

1. Epstein, Varda. "Nonverbal Learning Disorder: Is This What Your Child Has?" Kars4Kids, July 1, 2015.

2. Miller, Caroline. "What Is Nonverbal Learning Disorder?" Child Mind Institute, 2016.

3. Patino, Erica. "Understanding Nonverbal Learning Disabilities," Understood, May 21, 2014.

4. "Quick Facts On Nonverbal Learning Disorder," Child Mind Institute, 2016.

5. Thompson, Sue. "Nonverbal Learning Disorders," LDonline, 1996.

Chapter 14

Dyspraxia: Impaired Sensory And Motor Skills

Hearing or suspecting that your child may have dyspraxia can stir a lot of emotions. Even though dyspraxia is fairly common, many people have never heard of it.

Dyspraxia can affect a child's ability to do a wide range of everyday physical tasks. These can include things like jumping, speaking clearly and gripping a pencil. Some kids have mild symptoms and others more severe. There are lots of ways to help with dyspraxia at home and in school. Learning more about it can help you find the most effective solutions for your child.

What Is Dyspraxia?

Dyspraxia isn't a sign of muscle weakness or of low intelligence. It's a brain-based condition that makes it hard to plan and coordinate physical movement. Children with dyspraxia tend to struggle with balance and posture. They may appear clumsy or "out of sync" with their environment.

Dyspraxia goes by many names: developmental coordination disorder, motor learning difficulty, motor planning difficulty and apraxia of speech. It can affect the development of gross motor skills like walking or jumping. It can also affect fine motor skills. These include things like the hand movements needed to write clearly and the mouth and tongue movements needed to pronounce words correctly.

Dyspraxia can affect social skills too. Children with dyspraxia may behave immaturely even though they typically have average or above-average intelligence.

About This Chapter: Text in this chapter is excerpted from "Understanding Dyspraxia," © 2014–2016 Understood. org USA LLC. Reprinted with permission.

Kids don't outgrow dyspraxia. But occupational therapy, physical therapy, speech therapy and other tools and strategies can help. Kids can learn to work around areas of weakness and build on their strengths.

Different Kinds Of Dyspraxia

Dyspraxia can affect different kinds of movement. Professionals you speak to might break it down into these categories:

- **Ideomotor dyspraxia:** Makes it hard to complete single-step motor tasks such as combing hair and waving goodbye.

- **Ideational dyspraxia:** Makes it more difficult to perform a sequence of movements, like brushing teeth or making a bed.

- **Oromotor dyspraxia**, also called verbal apraxia or apraxia of speech: Makes it difficult to coordinate muscle movements needed to pronounce words. Kids with dyspraxia may have speech that is slurred and difficult to understand because they're unable to enunciate.

- **Constructional dyspraxia:** Makes it harder to understand spatial relationships. Kids with this type of dyspraxia may have difficulty copying geometric drawings or using building blocks.

How Common Is Dyspraxia?

Although dyspraxia isn't as widely discussed as other conditions that impact learning, like dyslexia, it's believed to be fairly common. Roughly 6 to 10 percent of children show some signs of dyspraxia.

Boys are affected more often than girls. But many people with symptoms are never diagnosed, prompting some experts to dub it a "hidden problem."

What Causes Dyspraxia?

Researchers don't know yet what causes dyspraxia. Many believe that genetics could play a role. Some scientists suspect dyspraxia may be caused by a problem with the nerve cells that send signals from the brain to muscles.

Researchers also believe that children who were born prematurely, had low birth weights or were exposed to alcohol in the womb may be more likely to have dyspraxia, though it's not clear why.

What Are The Symptoms Of Dyspraxia?

Dyspraxia affects some kids more severely than others. The signs you may be seeing can also look different as your child gets older. But generally, the symptoms are present early in life. Babies may be unusually irritable and have difficulties feeding. They may be slow to reach developmental milestones, such as rolling over or walking. Here are some common symptoms for different age groups. Some or all of these symptoms may be present.

Warning Signs in a Toddler

- Is a messy eater, preferring to eat with fingers rather than a fork or spoon

- Is unable to ride a tricycle or play ball

- Is delayed at becoming toilet trained

- Avoids playing with construction toys and puzzles

- Doesn't talk as well as kids the same age and might not say single words until age 3

Warning Signs in Preschool or Early Elementary School

- Often bumps into people and things

- Has trouble learning to jump and skip

- Is slow to develop left- or right-hand dominance

- Often drops objects or has difficulty holding them

- Has trouble grasping pencils and writing or drawing

- Has difficulty working buttons, snaps and zippers

- Speaks slowly or doesn't enunciate words

- Has trouble speaking at the right speed, volume and pitch

- Struggles to play and interact with other kids

Warning Signs in Grade School or Middle School

- Tries to avoid sports or gym class

- Takes a long time to write, due to difficulty gripping pencil and forming letters

- Has trouble moving objects from one place to another, such as pieces on a game board

- Struggles with games and activities that require hand-eye coordination

- Has trouble following instructions and remembering them

- Finds it difficult to stand for a long time as a result of weak muscle tone

Warning Signs in High School

- Has trouble with sports that involve jumping and cycling

- Tends to fall and trip; bumps into things and people

- May talk continuously and repeat things

- May forget and lose things

- Has trouble picking up on nonverbal signals from others

With treatment and support, children with dyspraxia may improve their muscle tone and coordination over time.

What Skills Are Affected By Dyspraxia?

Dyspraxia can affect a variety of skills. Here are some common ones. Keep in mind that there are ways to help your child improve in each of these areas:

- **Communication:** Kids with dyspraxia may struggle with different aspects of speech. They can have trouble pronouncing words or expressing their ideas. They may also have trouble adjusting the pitch and volume of their voice. As a result, making friends and being social can be much harder.

- **Emotional/behavioral skills:** Children with dyspraxia may behave immaturely. They may easily become overwhelmed in group settings. This can create problems with making friends, and kids can become anxious about socializing with others, especially as they get older. Their difficulties with sports may also affect their self-esteem and social abilities.

- **Academics:** Kids with dyspraxia often have difficulty writing quickly. This can create a number of classroom challenges, such as trouble taking notes and finishing tests. Children who have speech difficulties also may have difficulty with reading and spelling.

- **Overall life skills:** Dyspraxia can make it hard to master everyday tasks needed for independence. In elementary school, kids still may need help buttoning a shirt or brushing their teeth. As teens, they could have trouble learning to drive a car or fry an egg.

How Is Dyspraxia Diagnosed?

A good way to begin the diagnosis process is to start observing your child and taking notes on what you're seeing. To be diagnosed with dyspraxia, your child has to have symptoms for at least six months.

Taking notes can help you show that your child's behavior has been ongoing and is getting in the way of everyday tasks. This can make getting a diagnosis happen a little faster.

There's no one specific test to determine whether your child has dyspraxia. Typically, a doctor will examine your child to rule out other neurological conditions. Then your child may be referred to another professional. This could be a psychologist or an occupational therapist.

The specialist will interview you about what you've observed and test your child's strength, muscle tone and coordination. The specialist also will test your child's ability to carry out physical tasks, like throwing a ball. To diagnose your child with dyspraxia, the specialist needs to make four key findings:

- Motor skills lag behind what's expected based on the child's age.
- These difficulties interfere with the child's daily life or academic achievements.
- The weaknesses in motor skills aren't due to another neurological condition, such as cerebral palsy.
- Symptoms were present early in life, even though the condition typically isn't diagnosed before age 5.

If your child is diagnosed with dyspraxia, treatment can help. This might include occupational therapy or speech therapy. Getting a diagnosis can also help your child qualify for special supports and services in school, such as a laptop and word-prediction software to help with typing. Your child could also qualify for one-on-one time with a speech or occupational therapist.

What Conditions Are Related To Dyspraxia?

It's not unusual for children with dyspraxia to have other learning and attention issues. Doctors refer this to as comorbidity. If your child has dyspraxia, here are some other learning and attention issues you may want to read about:

- **Dyslexia:** Kids with dyslexia might have trouble learning to read. Dyslexia can also make it hard to write, spell and say the words you want to say.

- **Dyscalculia:** This causes kids to have difficulties with math. Kids with dyscalculia may have trouble remembering basic math facts such as 2 + 2 = 4, doing calculations and estimating quantities and times (such as how long a minute is). Dyspraxia can cause trouble with math, too.

- **Dysgraphia:** Dysgraphia causes trouble with writing. Dysgraphia and dyspraxia are very different, but they often have overlapping symptoms—like messy handwriting.

- **Attention-deficit hyperactivity disorder (ADHD):** ADHD can make it difficult for your child to keep still, concentrate, consider consequences and control impulses. About half of children with dyspraxia also have attention issues.

How Can Professionals Help With Dyspraxia?

Fortunately, there are many people who can help your child with dyspraxia. Some of these people may work in your child's school and some you might find in your community or online.

Therapists

A number of therapies can help with dyspraxia. Your child's teacher or doctor can help you find specialists who are trained in the following:

- **Occupational therapy:** An occupational therapist can help your child develop everyday skills needed to thrive in and out of school. This includes such things as learning to use a knife or write legibly.

- **Speech therapy:** A speech-language pathologist can pinpoint your child's speech issues and then suggest specific exercises that can help your child communicate more clearly.

- **Perceptual motor training:** This kind of training is typically done by occupational or physical therapists. It's designed to improve children's language, visual, movement and hearing and listening skills. It involves giving kids tasks to do that are challenging, but not so difficult that they become frustrated. Kids are given a series of exercises that will help them better learn how to integrate motor, sensory and language information.

Your Child's School

If your child has been diagnosed with dyspraxia and evaluated for special services, the school will come up with a plan of supports and accommodations, such as exempting your child from gym class. But even without a diagnosis, the school can do a number of things to help your child academically.

- Response to intervention (RTI) is a program that some schools use to screen students and provide extra help to those who are falling behind. If your child's school uses this program, then he may get small-group instruction in, say, writing or some other area. These small groups may meet in your child's regular classroom or in another part of the school. If your child doesn't make enough progress this way, the program will provide more intensive one-on-one instruction.

- Informal supports are strategies your child's teacher can use, such as breaking down writing assignments into "chunks," so that projects are more manageable for your child. The teacher may also let your child use a laptop in class if it's easier for him to type than to write things out by hand.

- If your child's teacher is using classroom accommodations, at some point you or the school may recommend getting a 504 plan for your child. This is a written plan that details how the school will accommodate your child's needs. Your child might get modified homework, extended time on tests and copies of all class notes.

- You may also want to consider requesting an evaluation for special education services. The evaluation will determine whether your child qualifies for an Individualized Education Program (IEP). This program can open the doors to even more resources, including assistive technology that your child can use at home and in school.

Parent Advocates

Every state has at least one Parent Training and Information Center or Community Parent Resource Center. These nonprofit centers are staffed by parents whose children have special needs. They know how to navigate the school system and can help you prepare for important school meetings and advocate for your child. You can find the center in your area through the Parent Technical Assistance Center Network's website.

What Can Be Done At Home For Dyspraxia?

You can do a lot to help your child with dyspraxia. Here are some strategies you may want to consider.

- **Learn as much as you can.** Dyspraxia isn't well known. Family, friends and even your child's teacher may not understand your child's struggles. Sharing information with them will enable you to help your child get the support he needs in and out of school.

- **Encourage physical activity.** Any kind of play that encourages physical activity will help your child develop motor skills. Whether it's a swim class or a simple game of hide-and-seek, it's good for a child with dyspraxia to get his body moving. It can also help your child build relationships with other kids.

- **Do jigsaw puzzles.** Puzzles can help your child work on visual or spatial perception. They can also help your child improve fine motor skills. Puzzles are fun for the whole family to do together.

- **Toss a bean bag.** This can be a fun way to help develop hand-eye coordination.

- **Get some pencil grips.** These inexpensive items can make writing easier. Give your child a variety of pens, including colored and scented markers, to help keep things interesting.

- **Practice keyboarding.** Typing may be easier for your child than handwriting. But it's a skill that needs to be learned and practiced.

- **Get some putty.** Squeezing Theraputty or some play-dough can help strengthen your child's hand muscles. It can also be a good stress reliever.

- **Download some apps.** Explore recommendations for fun apps that can help improve fine motor skills.

- **Adjust your expectations.** Your child may need help with grooming and other everyday activities long after peers have mastered those skills. By recognizing your child's challenges, you'll be able to give genuine praise when he completes these tasks.

- **Praise your child's efforts.** Reward your child for attempting a new task. Celebrate even the smallest bits of progress.

Dyspraxia can be very frustrating for your child and for you. But your child can succeed with the right tools and support. Having your love and encouragement will boost your child's self-esteem and help him stay motivated to keep trying hard.

Chapter 15
Information Processing Issues

If your child has a learning and attention issue, you may have heard the phrase *information processing issues*. That's not a diagnosis. It's a concept used in cognitive psychology as a way to understand several other learning issues. Here's what it means.

What Information Processing Is

When psychologists use this term, they're likening how the brain works to how a computer works. That includes how the mind collects information and how we use that data to do things.

We collect information in many ways, including through sight, smell, hearing, taste and touch. In computer terms, the information is known as *input*. But that's only the first step in information processing. Once we gather that data, our brain has to recognize, understand and store it.

Ultimately we have to respond to the information. That response is called *output*. Output is what we write, say, or do in reaction to the input.

Information processing covers the entire process. It's how the input and output work together. It's what makes it possible for kids to manage everything from reading a book to tying shoes.

What Information Processing Issues Are

Information processing issues arise when a child has trouble with either the input or the output—or both. Having these issues has nothing to do with the effort he's putting in. And it doesn't have anything to do with how smart he is.

Information processing issues *do* have to do with how the child's brain is recognizing and using the information it gets. Processing can affect many areas. But there are some critical ones that have to do with learning: visual processing and auditory processing.

Visual Information Processing Issues

Visual processing refers to how a child uses the data he sees. It involves how quickly he can understand something when he sees it and how well he remembers that information.

A child with visual information processing issues may have trouble accurately making sense of what he sees. He may lack visual-spatial skills. He may also:

- Find it hard to see the differences between similar-looking shapes or letters, like O and Q
- Have trouble comparing and seeing differences between certain colors, shapes and patterns
- Struggle to locate something specific on a page
- Skip lines when he reads or read the same line repeatedly
- Find it hard to stay in the lines when writing
- Have trouble copying information from the board
- Bump into things and have trouble navigating new places

Auditory Information Processing Issues

Auditory processing refers to how a child uses the data he hears. It involves how he makes sense of the sounds he's hearing and how he keeps up with the information.

A child with auditory information processing issues has trouble making sense of and getting meaning from what he hears. This is especially true when it's noisy. He may:

- Find it hard to tell the difference between similar-sounding words like *fifty* and *fifteen*
- Struggle to understand spoken language
- Have trouble following directions
- Find it hard to remember details he's heard
- Seem as though he's not listening

Not all kids with a certain kind of information processing issue will have the same difficulties. And a child who has an issue that involves information processing may also have trouble with working memory. Many kids also have a slower processing speed.

Finding Out If Your Child Has Trouble With Information Processing

If you think your child may have an information processing issue, the first step is to talk to his teacher. Discuss your concerns and ask what the teacher has noticed in class.

You might want to have your child evaluated to determine if one of these issues might be getting in the way of his learning. A full evaluation should include tests that look at processing skills. Testing can provide valuable information to help you and your child's teachers develop a plan to support his learning.

Chapter 16

Gifted Students With Learning Disabilities

How can a gifted student have a learning disability? At first glance, those seem like contradictory terms. And, indeed, when educators first began identifying a subgroup of students who exhibited both outstanding intellectual ability and learning disabilities, even some experts were skeptical. Yet research has found that about 14 percent of children classified as gifted might also have learning problems, compared to around 4 percent of all children.

But, unfortunately, not all teachers are trained to identify these co-occurring phenomena, and in some states programs are available to help either gifted children or those with learning disabilities, but not both. As a result, many students have been unable to get the specialized help they need. Luckily, the picture is changing as this issue is becoming better understood. More research is being done, new publications are appearing all the time, and many educational conferences now include sessions devoted to the topic.

> Gifted students may have underlying learning disabilities that include Asperger Syndrome, ADD (attention deficit disorder), ADHD (attention deficit hyperactivity disorder), and physical or emotional problems. In some cases when these disorders are identified, the student's gifted abilities may be overlooked.

Who Are Students With Learning Disabilities?

Gifted students with learning disabilities—often called "Gifted/LD," "double-labeled," or "twice exceptional" by educators—are those who exhibit extraordinary talent in some areas of

---

"Gifted Students With Learning Disabilities," © 2017 Omnigraphics. Reviewed December 2016.

academic achievement and disabling weaknesses in others. Because of their puzzling, inconsistent performance in school, they tend to be among the most misunderstood and misdiagnosed individuals in the student population, so they frequently fall through the cracks in the system and never get the type of attention they need. Many experts classify these students into three main groups:

- **Students who have been identified as gifted yet have difficulty at school.** These students have been identified as gifted by virtue of their IQ score, performance on standardized tests, or achievement in certain academic areas. But since they underperform in other areas, they are often mislabeled as "underachievers" or are simply called "lazy."

- **Those with an identified learning disability but whose intellectual ability has gone unnoticed.** Because this group of students struggle profoundly in school, their disability is readily apparent to educators and parents. But because efforts to help them focus only on correcting the disability, their talents may never be uncovered. As a result, their self-esteem suffers, they may become discouraged, and they might never reach their full potential in those areas in which they could succeed.

- **Students not classified as either gifted or learning disabled.** In a sense, these students' strengths and weaknesses cancel each other out, and they perform at an average grade level. Because they are doing well enough, their problems and abilities are not recognized, and they don't qualify for the special help they require in either area. Although grade-level performance may be adequate, this group of students has the potential for much higher achievement, but without the proper attention they might never get the chance to excel.

Identifying Students Who Are Both Gifted And Learning Disabled

Because the characteristics of Gifted/LD students vary from individual to individual, and because they are so often misunderstood, it can be difficult to identify them and address their needs. But there are a number of indicators they often have in common. A few of these include:

- Unexplained inconsistent academic performance.

- High achievement in complex interests outside of school.

- Excellent verbal skills but difficulty with written language.

- Difficulty with memorization but good at complex analysis.

- Excelling at one type of test (for example, multiple choice) but doing poorly on another.

- Wander off task frequently and daydream or become disruptive.

- Concentrate for long periods on tasks they find interesting but become bored when a subject doesn't interest them.

Helping Gifted Students With Learning Disabilities

The first steps in helping Gifted/LD students are to increase teacher education and community awareness and to expand special-needs programs to include curricula for these students. At the moment, many government and community programs do not include Gifted/LD children, and many school systems are not equipped to address their needs. Other suggestions include:

- Focus on the child's gift, not just the disability.

- Encourage students to choose tasks that rely on their strengths.

- Recognize and encourage individual learning styles.

- Stress concepts first, then details.

- Establish concrete goals, and celebrate successes.

- Provide accelerated coursework in gifted areas, remedial work for weak areas.

- Connect new lessons to past learning, and provide rationale for tasks.

- Help students develop compensation strategies for disabilities.

- Recognize student frustration, and allow them to withdraw from activities with dignity.

- Teach through discussion and inquiry, rather than rote memorization.

- Connect lessons to the world beyond the classroom.

- Establish individual, peer, and group counseling sessions.

- Promote self-awareness to help students develop their own learning strategies.

- Create a nurturing environment that values individual differences.

- Encourage interests outside of school that make use of special talents.

- Establish awareness, education, and support programs for parents, coaches, and other adults who are in regular contact with these students.

Gifted students with learning disabilities have the potential to achieve classroom success, become enthusiastic learners, develop self-confidence and gain the knowledge they need to be their own advocates throughout their lifetimes. But this will only happen through increased awareness on the part of teachers, parents, and the community, and through specialized educational programs designed to meet their needs.

References

1. Brody, Linda E. and Carol J. Mills. "Gifted Children with Learning Disabilities: A Review of the Issues," LDonline, 1997.

2. Douglass, Marcy J. "Twice Exceptional: Gifted Students with Learning Disabilities," WM.edu, May, 2007.

3. Perras, Cindy, M.Ed. "Gifted Students with LDs: What Teachers Need to Know," LDatSchool.ca, February 18, 2015.

4. Shenfield, Tali, C.Psych. "Helping Gifted Students with Learning Disability," Psy-Ed.com, October 18, 2016.

5. Wormald, Catherine. "Intellectually Gifted Students Often Have Learning Disabilities," TheConversation.com, March 24, 2015.

Part Three
Co-Occurring Disorders

Chapter 17
Attention Deficit Hyperactivity Disorder (ADHD)

Attention deficit hyperactivity disorder (ADHD) is a brain disorder marked by an ongoing pattern of inattention and/or hyperactivity-impulsivity that interferes with functioning or development.

- **Inattention** means a person wanders off task, lacks persistence, has difficulty sustaining focus, and is disorganized; and these problems are not due to defiance or lack of comprehension.

- **Hyperactivity** means a person seems to move about constantly, including in situations in which it is not appropriate; or excessively fidgets, taps, or talks. In adults, it may be extreme restlessness or wearing others out with constant activity.

- **Impulsivity** means a person makes hasty actions that occur in the moment without first thinking about them and that may have high potential for harm; or a desire for immediate rewards or inability to delay gratification. An impulsive person may be socially intrusive and excessively interrupt others or make important decisions without considering the long-term consequences.

Signs And Symptoms

Inattention and hyperactivity/impulsivity are the key behaviors of ADHD. Some people with ADHD only have problems with one of the behaviors, while others have both inattention and hyperactivity-impulsivity. Most children have the combined type of ADHD.

About This Chapter: This chapter includes text excerpted from "Attention Deficit Hyperactivity Disorder (ADHD)," National Institute of Mental Health (NIMH), March 2016.

In preschool, the most common ADHD symptom is hyperactivity.

It is normal to have some inattention, unfocused motor activity and impulsivity, but for people with ADHD, these behaviors:

- are more severe

- occur more often

- interfere with or reduce the quality of how they functions socially, at school, or in a job

Inattention

People with symptoms of inattention may often:

- Overlook or miss details, make careless mistakes in schoolwork, at work, or during other activities.

- Have problems sustaining attention in tasks or play, including conversations, lectures, or lengthy reading.

- Not seem to listen when spoken to directly.

- Not follow through on instructions and fail to finish schoolwork, chores, or duties in the workplace or start tasks but quickly lose focus and get easily sidetracked.

- Have problems organizing tasks and activities, such as what to do in sequence, keeping materials and belongings in order, having messy work and poor time management, and failing to meet deadlines.

- Avoid or dislike tasks that require sustained mental effort, such as schoolwork or homework, or for teens and older adults, preparing reports, completing forms or reviewing lengthy papers.

- Lose things necessary for tasks or activities, such as school supplies, pencils, books, tools, wallets, keys, paperwork, eyeglasses, and cell phones.

- Be easily distracted by unrelated thoughts or stimuli.

- Be forgetful in daily activities, such as chores, errands, returning calls, and keeping appointments.

Hyperactivity-Impulsivity

People with symptoms of hyperactivity-impulsivity may often:

- Fidget and squirm in their seats.

- Leave their seats in situations when staying seated is expected, such as in the classroom or in the office.

- Run or dash around or climb in situations where it is inappropriate or, in teens and adults, often feel restless.

- Be unable to play or engage in hobbies quietly.

- Be constantly in motion or "on the go," or act as if "driven by a motor."

- Talk nonstop.

- Blurt out an answer before a question has been completed, finish other people's sentences, or speak without waiting for a turn in conversation.

- Have trouble waiting his or her turn.

- Interrupt or intrude on others, for example in conversations, games, or activities.

Diagnosis of ADHD requires a comprehensive evaluation by a licensed clinician, such as a pediatrician, psychologist, or psychiatrist with expertise in ADHD. For a person to receive a diagnosis of ADHD, the symptoms of inattention and/or hyperactivity-impulsivity must be chronic or long-lasting, impair the person's functioning, and cause the person to fall behind normal development for his or her age. The doctor will also ensure that any ADHD symptoms are not due to another medical or psychiatric condition. Most children with ADHD receive a diagnosis during the elementary school years. For an adolescent or adult to receive a diagnosis of ADHD, the symptoms need to have been present prior to age 12.

ADHD symptoms can appear as early as between the ages of 3 and 6 and can continue through adolescence and adulthood. Symptoms of ADHD can be mistaken for emotional or disciplinary problems or missed entirely in quiet, well-behaved children, leading to a delay in diagnosis. Adults with undiagnosed ADHD may have a history of poor academic performance, problems at work, or difficult or failed relationships.

ADHD symptoms can change over time as a person ages. In young children with ADHD, hyperactivity-impulsivity is the most predominant symptom. As a child reaches elementary school, the symptom of inattention may become more prominent and cause the child to struggle academically. In adolescence, hyperactivity seems to lessen and may show more often as feelings of restlessness or fidgeting, but inattention and impulsivity may remain. Many adolescents with ADHD also struggle with relationships and antisocial behaviors. Inattention, restlessness, and impulsivity tend to persist into adulthood.

Risk Factors

Scientists are not sure what causes ADHD. Like many other illnesses, a number of factors can contribute to ADHD, such as:

- genes

- cigarette smoking, alcohol use, or drug use during pregnancy

- exposure to environmental toxins during pregnancy

- exposure to environmental toxins, such as high levels of lead, at a young age

- low birth weight

- brain injuries

ADHD is more common in males than females, and females with ADHD are more likely to have problems primarily with inattention. Other conditions, such as learning disabilities, anxiety disorder, conduct disorder, depression, and substance abuse, are common in people with ADHD.

Treatment And Therapies

While there is no cure for ADHD, currently available treatments can help reduce symptoms and improve functioning. Treatments include medication, psychotherapy, education or training, or a combination of treatments.

Medication

For many people, ADHD medications reduce hyperactivity and impulsivity and improve their ability to focus, work, and learn. Medication also may improve physical coordination. Sometimes several different medications or dosages must be tried before finding the right one that works for a particular person. Anyone taking medications must be monitored closely and carefully by their prescribing doctor.

Stimulants. The most common type of medication used for treating ADHD is called a "stimulant." Although it may seem unusual to treat ADHD with a medication that is considered a stimulant, it works because it increases the brain chemicals dopamine and norepinephrine, which play essential roles in thinking and attention.

Under medical supervision, stimulant medications are considered safe. However, there are risks and side effects, especially when misused or taken in excess of the prescribed dose. For example, stimulants can raise blood pressure and heart rate and increase anxiety. Therefore, a person with other health problems, including high blood pressure, seizures, heart disease, glaucoma, liver or kidney disease, or an anxiety disorder should tell their doctor before taking a stimulant.

Talk with a doctor if you see any of these side effects while taking stimulants:

- decreased appetite

- sleep problems

- tics (sudden, repetitive movements or sounds);

- personality changes

- increased anxiety and irritability

- stomachaches

- headaches

Nonstimulants. A few other ADHD medications are nonstimulants. These medications take longer to start working than stimulants, but can also improve focus, attention, and impulsivity in a person with ADHD. Doctors may prescribe a nonstimulant:

- when a person has bothersome side effects from stimulants;

- when a stimulant was not effective; or,

- in combination with a stimulant to increase effectiveness.

Although not approved by the U.S. Food and Drug Administration (FDA) specifically for the treatment of ADHD, some antidepressants are sometimes used alone or in combination with a stimulant to treat ADHD. Antidepressants may help all of the symptoms of ADHD and can be prescribed if a patient has bothersome side effects from stimulants. Antidepressants can be helpful in combination with stimulants if a patient also has another condition, such as an anxiety disorder, depression, or another mood disorder.

Doctors and patients can work together to find the best medication, dose, or medication combination.

Psychotherapy

Adding psychotherapy to treat ADHD can help patients and their families to better cope with everyday problems.

Behavioral therapy is a type of psychotherapy that aims to help a person change his or her behavior. It might involve practical assistance, such as help organizing tasks or completing schoolwork, or working through emotionally difficult events. Behavioral therapy also teaches a person how to:

- monitor his or her own behavior

- give oneself praise or rewards for acting in a desired way, such as controlling anger or thinking before acting

Parents, teachers, and family members also can give positive or negative feedback for certain behaviors and help establish clear rules, chore lists, and other structured routines to help a person control his or her behavior. Therapists may also teach children social skills, such as how to wait their turn, share toys, ask for help, or respond to teasing. Learning to read facial expressions and the tone of voice in others, and how to respond appropriately can also be part of social skills training.

Cognitive behavioral therapy can also teach a person mindfulness techniques, or meditation. A person learns how to be aware and accepting of one's own thoughts and feelings to improve focus and concentration. The therapist also encourages the person with ADHD to adjust to the life changes that come with treatment, such as thinking before acting, or resisting the urge to take unnecessary risks.

Family and marital therapy can help family members and spouses find better ways to handle disruptive behaviors, to encourage behavior changes, and improve interactions with the patient.

Education And Training

Children and adults with ADHD need guidance and understanding from their parents, families, and teachers to reach their full potential and to succeed. For school-age children, frustration, blame, and anger may have built up within a family before a child is diagnosed. Parents and children may need special help to overcome negative feelings. Mental health professionals can educate parents about ADHD and how it affects a family. They also will help the child and his or her parents develop new skills, attitudes, and ways of relating to each other.

Parenting skills training (behavioral parent management training) teaches parents the skills they need to encourage and reward positive behaviors in their children. It helps parents learn how to use a system of rewards and consequences to change a child's behavior. Parents are taught to give immediate and positive feedback for behaviors they want to encourage, and ignore or redirect behaviors that they want to discourage. They may also learn to structure situations in ways that support desired behavior.

Stress management techniques can benefit parents of children with ADHD by increasing their ability to deal with frustration so that they can respond calmly to their child's behavior.

Support groups can help parents and families connect with others who have similar problems and concerns. Groups often meet regularly to share frustrations and successes, to exchange information about recommended specialists and strategies, and to talk with experts.

Tips To Help Kids With ADHD Stay Organized

For Kids:

Parents and teachers can help kids with ADHD stay organized and follow directions with tools such as:

- **Keeping a routine and a schedule.** Keep the same routine every day, from wake-up time to bedtime. Include times for homework, outdoor play, and indoor activities. Keep the schedule on the refrigerator or on a bulletin board in the kitchen. Write changes on the schedule as far in advance as possible.

- **Organizing everyday items.** Have a place for everything, and keep everything in its place. This includes clothing, backpacks, and toys.

- **Using homework and notebook organizers.** Use organizers for school material and supplies. Stress to your child the importance of writing down assignments and bringing home the necessary books.

- **Being clear and consistent.** Children with ADHD need consistent rules they can understand and follow.

- **Giving praise or rewards when rules are followed.** Children with ADHD often receive and expect criticism. Look for good behavior, and praise it.

Chapter 18

Substance Abuse And Learning Disorders

You may have heard that teenagers with learning and attention issues are more likely to abuse alcohol and drugs than teens who don't have these issues. Do you have reason to be worried about your teen?

Not all teens with learning and attention issues will abuse drugs and alcohol. In fact, many don't. But it's important to understand the connection between learning and attention issues and substance abuse. Knowing how to identify signs of substance abuse is crucial for keeping your child healthy and safe.

Substance Abuse And Learning And Attention Issues: Likely Links

There are a number of studies that suggest teens with learning issues, such as dyslexia, and attention issues, such as attention-deficit hyperactivity disorder (ADHD), may be more likely to turn to substance abuse. There may be several reasons:

- Poor self-esteem
- Difficulties with schoolwork
- Loneliness
- Depression
- The desire to be accepted by peers

All these can affect teens with learning and attention issues. They're also factors that make teens more likely to abuse drugs and alcohol, according to the National Center on Addiction and Substance Abuse at Columbia University.

About This Chapter: Text in this chapter is excerpted from "The Truth About Learning And Attention Issues And Substance Abuse," © 2014–2016 Understood.org USA LLC. Reprinted with permission.

Research has found that teens with ADHD may be more likely to abuse alcohol, marijuana and cocaine than teens without ADHD. Some teens with ADHD may even become dependent on those substances.

Sometimes kids with ADHD have poor impulse control and want to do things that give them pleasure—even if those things are dangerous. And some teens turn to drugs in an effort to improve their attention spans or deal with the frustrations that can come from living with ADHD.

Possible Signs of Substance Abuse

It may not be obvious if your teen is abusing substances such as drugs or alcohol. Here are signs to watch for:

- Bloodshot eyes

- Pupils of eyes extremely small or large

- Secretive behavior; won't let you into the bedroom

- Change in group of friends

- Lying or stealing

- Loss of appetite (cocaine use)

- Increased appetite (marijuana use)

- Smell of alcohol on breath, or unusual-smelling breath (inhalant drugs)

- Sluggishness or constant sleeping

Some of these signs can also be due to emotional issues, such as depression or anxiety. Before you jump to any conclusions, talk to your teen. Encourage her to be honest with you about what's going on.

Treatment Reduces Risks

Perhaps the best way to prevent substance abuse problems is by helping your child find treatments for learning and attention issues. A child with ADHD might benefit from enrolling in a social skills class. Or you can check with your child's doctor to see if medication to treat ADHD is a good option.

Studies show that kids with ADHD who take medication for it are less likely to abuse substances and become dependent on them. That might be because teens who take ADHD medication have fewer ADHD symptoms, such as lack of impulse control.

Experts also think that if kids' learning and attention issues are treated when they're adolescents, they will be less likely to abuse substances as teens.

If you're concerned that your teen may be at risk for substance abuse, consider these ideas for reducing risky behavior (visit: www.understood.org/en/friends-feelings/teens-tweens/risky-behavior/7-ideas-for-reducing-risky-behaviors-in-teens), as well as resources for at-risk teens (visit: www.understood.org/en/friends-feelings/teens-tweens/risky-behavior/resources-for-parents-of-at-risk-teens).

How Does Drug Use Affect Your High School Grades?

Research shows that there is a definite link between teen substance abuse and how well you do in school. **Teens who abuse drugs have lower grades, a higher rate of absence from school and other activities, and an increased potential for dropping out of school.**

Although we all know or hear stories about people who use drugs and still get great grades, this is not typical. Most people who use drugs regularly don't consistently do well in school.

Studies show that marijuana, for example, affects your attention, memory, and ability to learn. Its effects can last for days or weeks after the drug wears off. So, if you are smoking marijuana daily, you are not functioning at your best.

Students who smoke marijuana tend to get lower grades and are more likely to drop out of high school. One marijuana study showed that heavy marijuana use in your teen years that continued into adulthood can reduce your IQ up to as much as 8 points.

(Source: "How Does Drug Use Affect Your High School Grades?" Just Think Twice, Drug Enforcement Administration (DEA).)

Chapter 19
Bipolar Disorder And Learning Disorders

What Is Bipolar Disorder?

Bipolar disorder is a serious brain illness. It is also called manic-depressive illness or manic depression. Children with bipolar disorder go through unusual mood changes. Sometimes they feel very happy or "up," and are much more energetic and active than usual, or than other kids their age. This is called a **manic episode.** Sometimes children with bipolar disorder feel very sad and "down," and are much less active than usual. This is called depression or a **depressive episode.**

Bipolar disorder is not the same as the normal ups and downs every kid goes through. Bipolar symptoms are more powerful than that. The mood swings are more extreme and are accompanied by changes in sleep, energy level, and the ability to think clearly. Bipolar symptoms are so strong, they can make it hard for a child to do well in school or get along with friends and family members. The illness can also be dangerous. Some young people with bipolar disorder try to hurt themselves or attempt suicide.

Children and teens with bipolar disorder should get treatment. With help, they can manage their symptoms and lead successful lives.

Who Develops Bipolar Disorder?

Anyone can develop bipolar disorder, including children and teens. However, most people with bipolar disorder develop it in their late teen or early adult years. The illness usually lasts a lifetime.

About This Chapter: This chapter includes text excerpted from "Bipolar Disorder In Children And Teens," National Institute of Mental Health (NIMH), 2015.

Why Does Someone Develop Bipolar Disorder?

Doctors do not know what causes bipolar disorder, but several things may contribute to the illness. Family genes may be one factor because bipolar disorder sometimes runs in families. However, it is important to know that just because someone in your family has bipolar disorder, it does not mean other members of the family will have it as well.

Another factor that may lead to bipolar disorder is the brain structure or the brain function of the person with the disorder. Scientists are finding out more about the disorder by studying it. This research may help doctors do a better job of treating people. Also, this research may help doctors to predict whether a person will get bipolar disorder. One day, doctors may be able to prevent the illness in some people.

What Are The Symptoms Of Bipolar Disorder?

Bipolar "mood episodes" include unusual mood changes along with unusual sleep habits, activity levels, thoughts, or behavior. In a child, these mood and activity changes must be very different from their usual behavior and from the behavior of other children. A person with bipolar disorder may have manic episodes, depressive episodes, or "mixed" episodes. A mixed episode has both manic and depressive symptoms. These mood episodes cause symptoms that last a week or two or sometimes longer. During an episode, the symptoms last every day for most of the day.

Children and teens having a manic episode may:

- feel very happy or act silly in a way that's unusual for them and for other people their age

- have a very short temper

- talk really fast about a lot of different things

- have trouble sleeping but not feel tired

- have trouble staying focused

- talk and think about sex more often

- do risky things

Children and teens having a depressive episode may:

- feel very sad

- complain about pain a lot, such as stomachaches and headaches

- sleep too little or too much

- feel guilty and worthless

- eat too little or too much

- have little energy and no interest in fun activities

- think about death or suicide

Can Children And Teens With Bipolar Disorder Have Other Problems?

Young people with bipolar disorder can have several problems at the same time. These include:

- **Substance abuse.** Both adults and kids with bipolar disorder are at risk of drinking or taking drugs.
- **Attention deficit hyperactivity disorder (ADHD).** Children who have both bipolar disorder and ADHD may have trouble staying focused.
- **Anxiety disorders**, like separation anxiety.

Sometimes behavior problems go along with mood episodes. Young people may take a lot of risks, such as driving too fast or spending too much money. Some young people with bipolar disorder think about suicide. **Watch for any signs of suicidal thinking. Take these signs seriously and call your child's doctor.**

How Is Bipolar Disorder Diagnosed?

An experienced doctor will carefully examine your child. There are no blood tests or brain scans that can diagnose bipolar disorder. Instead, the doctor will ask questions about your child's mood and sleeping patterns. The doctor will also ask about your child's energy and behavior. Sometimes doctors need to know about medical problems in your family, such as depression or alcoholism. The doctor may use tests to see if something other than bipolar disorder is causing your child's symptoms.

How Is Bipolar Disorder Treated?

Right now, there is no cure for bipolar disorder. Doctors often treat children who have the illness in much the same way they treat adults. Treatment can help control symptoms. Steady, dependable treatment works better than treatment that starts and stops. Treatment options include:

- **Medication.** There are several types of medication that can help. Children respond to medications in different ways, so the right type of medication depends on the child. Some children may need more than one type of medication because their symptoms are so complex. Sometimes they need to try different types of medicine to see which are best for them. Children should take the fewest number of medications and the smallest doses possible to help their symptoms. A good way to remember this is "start low, go slow."

- **Therapy.** Different kinds of psychotherapy, or "talk" therapy, can help children with bipolar disorder. Therapy can help children change their behavior and manage their routines. It can also help young people get along better with family and friends. Sometimes therapy includes family members.

> Medications can cause side effects. **Always tell your child's doctor about any problems with side effects.** Do not stop giving your child medication without a doctor's help. Stopping medication suddenly can be dangerous, and it can make bipolar symptoms worse.

What Can Children And Teens Expect From Treatment?

With treatment, children and teens with bipolar disorder can get better over time. It helps when doctors, parents, and young people work together.

Sometimes a child's bipolar disorder changes. When this happens, treatment needs to change too. For example, your child may need to try a different medication. The doctor may also recommend other treatment changes. Symptoms may come back after a while, and more adjustments may be needed. Treatment can take time, but sticking with it helps many children and teens have fewer bipolar symptoms.

You can help treatment be more effective. Try keeping a chart of your child's moods, behaviors, and sleep patterns. This is called a "daily life chart" or "mood chart." It can help you and your child understand and track the illness. A chart can also help the doctor see whether treatment is working.

Personal Story

James has bipolar disorder.

Here's his story.

Four months ago, James found out he has bipolar disorder. He knows it's a serious illness, but he was relieved when he found out. That's because he had symptoms for years, but no one knew what was wrong. Now he's getting treatment and feeling better.

James often felt really sad. As a kid, he skipped school or stayed in bed when he was down. At other times, he felt really happy. He talked fast and felt like he could do anything. James lived like this for a long time, but things changed last year. His job got very stressful. He felt like he was having more "up" and "down" times. His wife and friends wanted to know what was wrong. He told them to leave him alone and said everything was fine.

A few weeks later, James couldn't get out of bed. He felt awful, and the bad feelings went on for days. Then, his wife took him to the family doctor, who sent James to a psychiatrist. He talked to this doctor about how he was feeling. Soon James could see that his ups and downs were serious. He was diagnosed with bipolar disorder, and he started treatment.

These days, James takes medicine and goes to talk therapy. Treatment was hard at first, and recovery took some time, but now he's back at work. His mood changes are easier to handle, and he's having fun again with his wife and friends.

(Source: "Bipolar Disorder," National Institute of Mental Health (NIMH).)

How Does Bipolar Disorder Affect Parents And Family?

Taking care of a child or teenager with bipolar disorder can be stressful for you, too. You have to cope with the mood swings and other problems, such as short tempers and risky activities. This can challenge any parent. Sometimes the stress can strain your relationships with other people, and you may miss work or lose free time.

If you are taking care of a child with bipolar disorder, take care of yourself too. Find someone you can talk to about your feelings. Talk with the doctor about support groups for caregivers. If you keep your stress level down, you will do a better job. It might help your child get better too.

I Know Someone Who Is In Crisis. What Do I Do?

If you know someone who might be thinking about hurting himself or herself or someone else, get help quickly.

- Do not leave the person alone.

- Call your doctor.

- Call 911 or go to the emergency room.

- Call National Suicide Prevention Lifeline, toll-free: 800-273-TALK (800-273-8255). The TTY number is 800-799-4TTY (800-799-4889).

Chapter 20
Conduct Disorder Often Associated With Attention Deficit Disorder

Attention deficit hyperactivity disorder (ADHD) often occurs with other disorders. About half of children with ADHD referred to clinics have other disorders as well as ADHD.

The combination of ADHD with other disorders often presents extra challenges for children, parents, educators, and healthcare providers. Therefore, it is important for doctors to screen every child with ADHD for other disorders and problems. This chapter provides an overview of the more common conditions and concerns that can occur with ADHD. Talk with your doctor if you have concerns about your child's symptoms.

Behavior Or Conduct Problems

Children occasionally act angry or defiant around adults or respond aggressively when they are upset. When these behaviors persist over time, or are severe, they can become a behavior disorder. Children with ADHD are more likely to be diagnosed with a behavior disorder such as Oppositional Defiant Disorder or Conduct Disorder. About 1 in 4 children with ADHD have a diagnosed behavior disorder.

Oppositional Defiant Disorder (ODD)

When children act out persistently so that it causes serious problems at home, in school, or with peers, they may be diagnosed with ODD. ODD is one of the most common disorders occurring with ADHD. ODD usually starts before 8 years of age, but can also occur in

About This Chapter: Text in this chapter begins with excerpts from "Attention-Deficit / Hyperactivity Disorder (ADHD)," Centers for Disease Control and Prevention (CDC), October 5, 2016; Text beginning with the heading "Managing Symptoms: Staying Healthy" is excerpted from "Children's Mental Health," Centers for Disease Control and Prevention (CDC), November 16, 2016.

adolescents. Children with ODD may be most likely to act oppositional or defiant around people they know well, such as family members or a regular care provider. Children with ODD show these behaviors more often than other children their age.

Examples of ODD behaviors include:

- often losing their temper

- arguing with adults or refusing to comply with adults' rules or requests

- often getting angry, being resentful, or wanting to hurt someone who they feel has hurt them or caused problems for them

- deliberately annoying others; easily becoming annoyed with others

- often blaming other people for their own mistakes or misbehavior

> - The average prevalence of ODD is estimated at 3.3 percent, and occurs more often in boys than girls.
> - Children who experienced harsh, inconsistent, or neglectful child-rearing practices are at increased risk for developing ODD.
>
> *(Source: "Mental Disorders," Substance Abuse and Mental Health Services Administration (SAMHSA).)*

Conduct Disorder (CD)

CD is diagnosed when children show a behavioral pattern of aggression toward others, and serious violations of rules and social norms at home, in school, and with peers. These behaviors often lead to breaking the law and being jailed. Having ADHD makes a child more likely to be diagnosed with CD. Children with CD are more likely to get injured, and have difficulties getting along with peers.

Examples of CD behaviors include

- breaking serious rules, such as running away, staying out at night when told not to, or skipping school

- being aggressive in a way that causes harm, such as bullying, fighting, or being cruel to animals

- lying and stealing, or damaging other people's property on purpose

An estimated 8.5 percent of children and youth meet criteria for conduct disorder at some point in their life. Prevalence increases from childhood to adolescence and is more common among males than females.

Conduct disorder may be preceded by temperamental risk factors, such as behavioral difficulties in infancy and below-average intelligence. Similar to ODD, environmental risk factors may include harsh or inconsistent child-rearing practices and/or child maltreatment. Parental criminality, frequent changes of caregivers, large family size, familial psychopathology, and early institutional living may also contribute to risk for developing the disorder. Community-level risk factors may include neighborhood exposure to violence, peer rejection, and association with a delinquent peer group. Children with a parent or sibling with conduct disorder or other behavioral health disorders (for example, ADHD, schizophrenia, severe alcohol use disorder) are more likely to develop the condition. Children with conduct disorder often present with other disorders as well, including ADHD, learning disorders, and depression.

(Source: "Mental Disorders," Substance Abuse and Mental Health Services Administration (SAMHSA).)

Treatment For Disruptive Behavior Disorders

Starting treatment early is important. Treatment is most effective if it fits the needs of the child and family. The first step to treatment is to have a comprehensive evaluation by a mental health professional. Some of the signs of behavior problems, such as not following rules, are also signs of ADHD, so it is important to get a careful evaluation to see if a child has both conditions. For younger children, the treatment with the strongest evidence is behavioral parent training, where a therapist helps the parent learn effective ways to strengthen the parent-child relationship and respond to the child's behavior. For school-age children and teens, an often-used effective treatment is combination training and therapy that includes the child, the family, and the school. Sometimes medication is part of the treatment.

Managing Symptoms: Staying Healthy

Being healthy is important for all children and can be especially important for children with behavior or conduct problems. In addition to behavioral therapy and medication, practicing certain healthy lifestyle behaviors may reduce challenging and disruptive behaviors your child might experience. Here are some healthy behaviors that may help:

- Engaging in regular physical activity, including aerobic and vigorous exercise.

- Eating a healthful diet centered on fruits, vegetables, whole grains, legumes (for example, beans, peas, and lentils), lean protein sources, and nuts and seeds.

- Getting the recommended amount of sleep each night based on age.

- Strengthening relationships with family members.

Prevention Of Disruptive Behavior Disorders

It is not known exactly why some children develop disruptive behavior disorders. Many factors may play a role, including biological and social factors. It is known that children are at greater risk when they are exposed to other types of violence and criminal behavior, when they experience maltreatment or harsh or inconsistent parenting, or when their parents have mental health conditions like substance use disorders, depression, or ADHD. The quality of early childhood care also can impact whether a child develops behavior problems.

Although these factors appear to increase the risk for disruptive behavior disorders, there are ways to decrease the chance that children experience them.

Part Four
Other Disabilities And Chronic
Conditions That Affect Learning

Chapter 21

Cancer Treatment Associated With Learning Disabilities

The treatment of cancer may cause health problems for childhood cancer survivors months or years after successful treatment has ended. Cancer treatments may harm the body's organs, tissues, or bones and cause health problems later in life. These health problems are called late effects.

Treatments that may cause late effects include the following:

- surgery
- chemotherapy
- radiation therapy
- stem cell transplant

Doctors are studying the late effects caused by cancer treatment. They are working to improve cancer treatments and stop or lessen late effects. While most late effects are not life-threatening, they may cause serious problems that affect health and quality of life.

Late Effects In Childhood Cancer Survivors

Late effects in childhood cancer survivors may affect the following:

- organs, tissues, and body function.
- growth and development.
- mood, feelings, and actions.

About This Chapter: This chapter includes text excerpted from "Late Effects Of Treatment For Childhood Cancer (PDQ®)—Patient Version," National Cancer Institute (NCI), August 11, 2016.

- thinking, learning, and memory.

- social and psychological adjustment.

- risk of second cancers.

Cognitive Late Effects Of Childhood Cancer Treatment

Cognitive late effects include changes in your child's ability to memorize, learn, and think. These types of late effects are more likely to occur in children who've had certain cancers such as brain and spinal cord tumors, head and neck cancers, and some types of leukemia, such as acute lymphoblastic leukemia (ALL). Treatments such as radiation therapy to the head and certain types of chemotherapy also increase the risk of cognitive late effects. These late effects are also more likely in children who were very young during treatment, who received very high doses of treatment, and whose treatment lasted for a long time.

Children with cognitive late effects may have a more difficult time:

- memorizing or remembering
- learning (handwriting, spelling, reading, vocabulary, and/or math may be particularly challenging)
- thinking (including concentrating, completing work on time, doing work that involves multiple steps, problem solving, and planning)

(Source: "Coping With Cancer: Survivorship Care For Children," National Cancer Institute (NCI).)

Important Factors That Affect The Risk Of Late Effects

Many childhood cancer survivors will have late effects. The risk of late effects depends on factors related to the tumor, treatment, and patient. These include the following:

1. Tumor-related factors:

   - Type of cancer.

   - Where the tumor is in the body.

   - How the tumor affects the way tissues and organs work.

2. Treatment-related factors:

   - Type of surgery.

- Chemotherapy type, dose, and schedule.

- Type of radiation therapy, part of the body treated, and dose.

- Stem cell transplant.

- Use of two or more types of treatment at the same time.

- Blood product transfusion.

- Chronic graft-versus-host disease.

3. Patient-related factors:

- The child's gender.

- Health problems the child had before being diagnosed with cancer.

- The child's age and developmental stage when diagnosed and treated.

- Length of time since diagnosis and treatment.

- Changes in hormone levels.

- The ability of healthy tissue affected by cancer treatment to repair itself.

- Certain changes in the child's genes.

- Family history of cancer or other conditions.

- Health habits.

The chance of having late effects increases over time.

New treatments for childhood cancer have decreased the number of deaths from the primary cancer. Because childhood cancer survivors are living longer, they are having more late effects after cancer treatment. Survivors may not live as long as people who did not have cancer. The most common causes of death in childhood cancer survivors are:

- The primary cancer comes back.

- A second (different) primary cancer forms.

- Heart and lung damage.

Studies of the causes of late effects have led to changes in treatment. This has improved the quality of life for cancer survivors and helps prevent illness and death from late effects.

Follow-Up Care

Regular follow-up by health professionals who are trained to find and treat late effects is important for the long-term health of childhood cancer survivors. Follow-up care will be different for each person who has been treated for cancer. The type of care will depend on the type of cancer, the type of treatment, genetic factors, and the person's general health and health habits. Follow-up care includes checking for signs and symptoms of late effects and health education on how to prevent or lessen late effects.

It is important that childhood cancer survivors have an exam at least once a year. The exams should be done by a health professional who knows the survivor's risk for late effects and can recognize the early signs of late effects. Blood and imaging tests may also be done.

Long-term follow-up may improve the health and quality of life for cancer survivors. It also helps doctors study the late effects of cancer treatments so that safer therapies for newly diagnosed children may be developed.

Good health habits are also important for survivors of childhood cancer.

The quality of life for cancer survivors may be improved by behaviors that promote health and well-being. These include a healthy diet, exercise, and regular medical and dental checkups. These self-care behaviors are especially important for cancer survivors because of their risk of health problems related to treatment. Healthy behaviors may make late effects less severe and lower the risk of other diseases.

Avoiding behaviors that are damaging to health is also important. Smoking, excess alcohol use, illegal drug use, being exposed to sunlight, or not being physically active may worsen organ damage related to treatment and may increase the risk of second cancers.

Chapter 22
Aphasia

What Is Aphasia?

Aphasia is a disorder that results from damage to portions of the brain that are responsible for language. For most people, these areas are on the left side of the brain. Aphasia usually occurs suddenly, often following a stroke or head injury, but it may also develop slowly, as the result of a brain tumor or a progressive neurological disease. The disorder impairs the expression and understanding of language as well as reading and writing. Aphasia may co-occur with speech disorders, such as dysarthria or apraxia of speech, which also result from brain damage.

Who Can Acquire Aphasia?

Most people who have aphasia are middle-aged or older, but anyone can acquire it, including young children. About 1 million people in the United States currently have aphasia, and nearly 180,000 Americans acquire it each year, according to the National Aphasia Association (NAA).

What Causes Aphasia?

Aphasia is caused by damage to one or more of the language areas of the brain. Most often, the cause of the brain injury is a stroke. A stroke occurs when a blood clot or a leaking or burst vessel cuts off blood flow to part of the brain. Brain cells die when they do not receive their normal supply of blood, which carries oxygen and important nutrients. Other causes of brain injury are severe blows to the head, brain tumors, gunshot wounds, brain infections, and progressive neurological disorders, such as Alzheimer disease.

About This Chapter: This chapter includes text excerpted from "Aphasia," National Institute on Deafness and Other Communication Disorders (NIDCD), June 1, 2016.

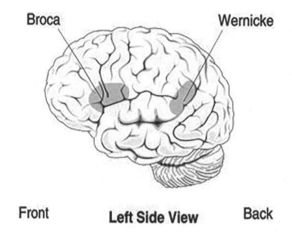

Figure 22.1. Areas Of The Brain Affected By Broca And Wernicke Aphasia

What Types Of Aphasia Are There?

There are two broad categories of aphasia: fluent and nonfluent, and there are several types within these groups.

Damage to the temporal lobe of the brain may result in **Wernicke aphasia** (see Figure 22.1), the most common type of fluent aphasia. People with Wernicke aphasia may speak in long, complete sentences that have no meaning, adding unnecessary words and even creating made-up words.

For example, someone with Wernicke aphasia may say, "You know that smoodle pinkered and that I want to get him round and take care of him like you want before."

As a result, it is often difficult to follow what the person is trying to say. People with Wernicke aphasia are often unaware of their spoken mistakes. Another hallmark of this type of aphasia is difficulty understanding speech.

The most common type of nonfluent aphasia is **Broca aphasia** (see Figure 22.1). People with Broca aphasia have damage that primarily affects the frontal lobe of the brain. They often have right-sided weakness or paralysis of the arm and leg because the frontal lobe is also important for motor movements. People with Broca aphasia may understand speech and know what they want to say, but they frequently speak in short phrases that are produced with great effort. They often omit small words, such as "is," "and" and "the."

For example, a person with Broca aphasia may say, "Walk dog," meaning, "I will take the dog for a walk," or "book book two table," for "There are two books on the table." People with

Broca aphasia typically understand the speech of others fairly well. Because of this, they are often aware of their difficulties and can become easily frustrated.

Another type of aphasia, **global aphasia**, results from damage to extensive portions of the language areas of the brain. Individuals with global aphasia have severe communication difficulties and may be extremely limited in their ability to speak or comprehend language. They may be unable to say even a few words or may repeat the same words or phrases over and over again. They may have trouble understanding even simple words and sentences.

There are other types of aphasia, each of which results from damage to different language areas in the brain. Some people may have difficulty repeating words and sentences even though they understand them and can speak fluently (conduction aphasia). Others may have difficulty naming objects even though they know what the object is and what it may be used for (anomic aphasia).

Sometimes, blood flow to the brain is temporarily interrupted and quickly restored. When this type of injury occurs, which is called a transient ischemic attack, language abilities may return in a few hours or days.

How Is Aphasia Diagnosed?

Aphasia is usually first recognized by the physician who treats the person for his or her brain injury. Most individuals will undergo a magnetic resonance imaging (MRI) or computed tomography (CT) scan to confirm the presence of a brain injury and to identify its precise location. The physician also typically tests the person's ability to understand and produce language, such as following commands, answering questions, naming objects, and carrying on a conversation.

If the physician suspects aphasia, the patient is usually referred to a speech-language pathologist, who performs a comprehensive examination of the person's communication abilities. The person's ability to speak, express ideas, converse socially, understand language, and read and write are all assessed in detail.

How Is Aphasia Treated?

Following a brain injury, tremendous changes occur in the brain, which help it to recover. As a result, people with aphasia often see dramatic improvements in their language and communication abilities in the first few months, even without treatment. But in many cases, some aphasia remains following this initial recovery period. In these instances, speech-language therapy is used to help patients regain their ability to communicate.

Research has shown that language and communication abilities can continue to improve for many years and are sometimes accompanied by new activity in brain tissue near the damaged area. Some of the factors that may influence the amount of improvement include the cause of the brain injury, the area of the brain that was damaged and its extent, and the age and health of the individual.

Aphasia therapy aims to improve a person's ability to communicate by helping him or her to use remaining language abilities, restore language abilities as much as possible, and learn other ways of communicating, such as gestures, pictures, or use of electronic devices. Individual therapy focuses on the specific needs of the person, while group therapy offers the opportunity to use new communication skills in a small-group setting.

Recent technologies have provided new tools for people with aphasia. "Virtual" speech pathologists provide patients with the flexibility and convenience of getting therapy in their homes through a computer. The use of speech-generating applications on mobile devices like tablets can also provide an alternative way to communicate for people who have difficulty using spoken language.

Increasingly, patients with aphasia participate in activities, such as book clubs, technology groups, and art and drama clubs. Such experiences help patients regain their confidence and social self-esteem, in addition to improving their communication skills. Stroke clubs, regional support groups formed by people who have had a stroke, are available in most major cities. These clubs can help a person and his or her family adjust to the life changes that accompany stroke and aphasia.

Family involvement is often a crucial component of aphasia treatment because it enables family members to learn the best way to communicate with their loved one.

Family members are encouraged to:

- Participate in therapy sessions, if possible.

- Simplify language by using short, uncomplicated sentences.

- Repeat the content words or write down key words to clarify meaning as needed.

- Maintain a natural conversational manner appropriate for an adult.

- Minimize distractions, such as a loud radio or TV, whenever possible.

- Include the person with aphasia in conversations.

- Ask for and value the opinion of the person with aphasia, especially regarding family matters.

- Encourage any type of communication, whether it is speech, gesture, pointing, or drawing.

- Avoid correcting the person's speech.

- Allow the person plenty of time to talk.

- Help the person become involved outside the home. Seek out support groups, such as stroke clubs.

What Research Is Being Done For Aphasia?

Researchers are testing new types of speech-language therapy in people with both recent and chronic aphasia to see if new methods can better help them recover word retrieval, grammar, prosody (tone), and other aspects of speech.

Some of these new methods involve improving cognitive abilities that support the processing of language, such as short-term memory and attention. Others involve activities that stimulate the mental representations of sounds, words, and sentences, making them easier to access and retrieve.

Researchers are also exploring drug therapy as an experimental approach to treating aphasia. Some studies are testing whether drugs that affect the chemical neurotransmitters in the brain can be used in combination with speech-language therapy to improve recovery of various language functions.

Other research is focused on using advanced imaging methods, such as functional magnetic resonance imaging (fMRI), to explore how language is processed in the normal and damaged brain and to understand recovery processes. This type of research may advance our knowledge of how the areas involved in speech and understanding language reorganize after a brain injury. The results could have implications for the diagnosis and treatment of aphasia and other neurological disorders.

A relatively new area of interest in aphasia research is noninvasive brain stimulation in combination with speech-language therapy. Two such brain stimulation techniques, transcranial magnetic stimulation (TMS) and transcranial direct current stimulation (tDCS), temporarily alter normal brain activity in the region being stimulated.

Researchers originally used these techniques to help them understand the parts of the brain that played a role in language and recovery after a stroke. Recently, scientists are studying if this temporary alteration of brain activity might help people re-learn language use.

Chapter 23

Cerebral Palsy Often Connected To A Learning Disability

What Is Cerebral Palsy?

Cerebral palsy (CP) refers to a group of neurological disorders that appear in infancy or early childhood and permanently affect body movement and muscle coordination CP is caused by damage to or abnormalities inside the developing brain that disrupt the brain's ability to control movement and maintain posture and balance. The term cerebral refers to the brain; palsy refers to the loss or impairment of motor function.

CP affects the motor area of the brain's outer layer (called the cerebral cortex), the part of the brain that directs muscle movement.

In some cases, the cerebral motor cortex hasn't developed normally during fetal growth. In others, the damage is a result of injury to the brain either before, during, or after birth. In either case, the damage is not repairable and the disabilities that result are permanent.

Children with CP exhibit a wide variety of symptoms, including:

- lack of muscle coordination when performing voluntary movements (ataxia);
- stiff or tight muscles and exaggerated reflexes (spasticity);
- weakness in one or more arm or leg;
- walking on the toes, a crouched gait, or a "scissored" gait;
- variations in muscle tone, either too stiff or too floppy;

About This Chapter: This chapter includes text excerpted from "Cerebral Palsy: Hope Through Research," National Institute of Neurological Disorders and Stroke (NINDS), November 2, 2016.

- excessive drooling or difficulties swallowing or speaking;

- shaking (tremor) or random involuntary movements;

- delays in reaching motor skill milestones; and

- difficulty with precise movements such as writing or buttoning a shirt.

> The symptoms of CP differ in type and severity from one person to the next, and may even change in an individual over time. Symptoms may vary greatly among individuals, depending on which parts of the brain have been injured. All people with CP have problems with movement and posture, and some also have some level of intellectual disability, seizures, and abnormal physical sensations or perceptions, as well as other medical disorders. People with CP also may have impaired vision or hearing, and language, and speech problems.

CP is the leading cause of childhood disabilities, but it doesn't always cause profound disabilities. While one child with severe CP might be unable to walk and need extensive, lifelong care, another child with mild CP might be only slightly awkward and require no special assistance. The disorder isn't progressive, meaning it doesn't get worse over time. However, as the child gets older, certain symptoms may become more or less evident.

A study by the Centers for Disease Control and Prevention (CDC) shows the average prevalence of CP is 3.3 children per 1,000 live births.

There is no cure for CP, but supportive treatments, medications, and surgery can help many individuals improve their motor skills and ability to communicate with the world.

What Causes Cerebral Palsy?

CP is caused by abnormal development of part of the brain or by damage to parts of the brain that control movement. This damage can occur before, during, or shortly after birth. The majority of children have congenital CP (that is, they were born with it), although it may not be detected until months or years later. A small number of children have acquired CP, which means the disorder begins after birth. Some causes of acquired CP include brain damage in the first few months or years of life, brain infections such as bacterial meningitis or viral encephalitis, problems with blood flow to the brain, or head injury from a motor vehicle accident, a fall, or child abuse.

In many cases, the cause of CP is unknown. Possible causes include genetic abnormalities, congenital brain malformations, maternal infections or fevers, or fetal injury, for example. The following types of brain damage may cause its characteristic symptoms:

- damage to the white matter of the brain (periventricular leukomalacia, or PVL)

- abnormal development of the brain (cerebral dysgenesis)

- bleeding in the brain (intracranial hemorrhage)

- severe lack of oxygen in the brain (asphyxia)

What Are The Different Forms?

The specific forms of CP are determined by the extent, type, and location of a child's abnormalities. Doctors classify CP according to the type of movement disorder involved—*spastic* (stiff muscles), *athetoid* (writhing movements), or *ataxic* (poor balance and coordination)—plus any additional symptoms, such weakness (*paresis*) or paralysis (*plegia*). For example, *hemiparesis* (hemi = half) indicates that only one side of the body is weakened. *Quadriplegia* (quad = four) means all four limbs are affected.

Spastic CP is the most common type of the disorder. People have stiff muscles and awkward movements. Forms of spastic CP include:

- *Spastic hemiplegia/hemiparesis* typically affects the arm and hand on one side of the body, but it can also include the leg. Some children will develop an abnormal curvature of the spine (scoliosis). A child with spastic hemiplegia may also have seizures. Speech will be delayed and, at best, may be competent, but intelligence is usually normal.

- *Spastic diplegia/diparesis* involves muscle stiffness that is predominantly in the legs and less severely affects the arms and face, although the hands may be clumsy. Intelligence and language skills are usually normal.

- *Spastic quadriplegia/quadriparesis* is the most severe form of CP and is often associated with moderate-to-severe intellectual disability. It is caused by widespread damage to the brain or significant brain malformations. Children will often have severe stiffness in their limbs but a floppy neck. They are rarely able to walk. Speaking and being understood are difficult. Seizures can be frequent and hard to control.

Dyskinetic CP (also includes athetoid, choreoathetoid, and dystonic CP) is characterized by slow and uncontrollable writhing or jerky movements of the hands, feet, arms, or legs. Some children have problems hearing, controlling their breathing, and/or coordinating the muscle movements required for speaking. Intelligence is rarely affected in these forms of CP.

Ataxic CP affects balance and depth perception. Children with ataxic CP will often have poor coordination and walk unsteadily with a wide-based gait.

Mixed types of CP refer to symptoms that don't correspond to any single type of CP but are a mix of types. For example, a child with mixed CP may have some muscles that are too tight and others that are too relaxed, creating a mix of stiffness and floppiness.

What Other Conditions Are Associated With Cerebral Palsy?

Intellectual disability. Approximately 30–50 percent of individuals with CP will be intellectually impaired. Mental impairment is more common among those with spastic quadriplegia than in those with other types of CP.

Learning difficulties. Children with CP may have difficulty processing particular types of spatial and auditory information. Brain damage may affect the development of language and intellectual functioning.

Speech and language disorders. Speech and language disorders, such as difficulty forming words and speaking clearly, are present in more than a third of persons with CP. Poor speech impairs communication and is often interpreted as a sign of cognitive impairment, which can be very frustrating to children with CP, especially the majority who have average to above average intelligence,

Impaired vision. Many children with CP have strabismus, commonly called "cross eyes," which left untreated can lead to poor vision in one eye and can interfere with the ability to judge distance. Some children with CP have difficulty understanding and organizing visual information. Other children may have defective vision or blindness that blurs the normal field of vision in one or both eyes.

Hearing loss. Impaired hearing is also more frequent among those with CP than in the general population. Some children have partial or complete hearing loss, particularly as the result of jaundice or lack of oxygen to the developing brain.

Seizure disorder. As many as half of all children with CP have one or more seizures. Children with both CP and epilepsy are more likely to have intellectual disability.

Delayed growth and development. Children with moderate to severe CP, especially those with spastic quadriparesis, often lag behind in growth and development. In babies this lag usually takes the form of too little weight gain. In young children it can appear as abnormal shortness, and in teenagers it may appear as a combination of shortness and lack of sexual development. The muscles and limbs affected by CP tend to be smaller than normal, especially in children with spastic hemiplegia, whose limbs on the affected side of the body may not grow as quickly or as long as those on the normal side.

Spinal deformities and osteoarthritis. Deformities of the spine—curvature (scoliosis), humpback (kyphosis), and saddle back (lordosis)—are associated with CP. Spinal deformities can make sitting, standing, and walking difficult and cause chronic back pain. Pressure on and misalignment of the joints may result in osteoporosis (a breakdown of cartilage in the joints and bone enlargement).

Drooling. Some individuals with CP drool because they have poor control of the muscles of the throat, mouth, and tongue.

Incontinence. A possible complication of CP is incontinence, caused by poor control of the muscles that keep the bladder closed.

Abnormal sensations and perceptions. Some individuals with CP experience pain or have difficulty feeling simple sensations, such as touch.

Infections and long-term illnesses. Many adults with CP have a higher risk of heart and lung disease, and pneumonia (often from inhaling bits of food into the lungs), than those without the disorder.

Contractures. Muscles can become painfully fixed into abnormal positions, called contractures, which can increase muscle spasticity and joint deformities in people with CP.

Malnutrition. Swallowing, sucking, or feeding difficulties can make it difficult for many individuals with CP, particularly infants, to get proper nutrition and gain or maintain weight.

Dental problems. Many children with CP are at risk of developing gum disease and cavities because of poor dental hygiene. Certain medications, such as seizure drugs, can exacerbate these problems.

Inactivity. Childhood inactivity is magnified in children with CP due to impairment of the motor centers of the brain that produce and control voluntary movement. While children with CP may exhibit increased energy expenditure during activities of daily living, movement impairments make it difficult for them to participate in sports and other activities at a level of intensity sufficient to develop and maintain strength and fitness. Inactive adults with disability exhibit increased severity of disease and reduced overall health and well-being.

How Is Cerebral Palsy Treated?

CP can't be cured, but treatment will often improve a child's capabilities. Many children go on to enjoy near-normal adult lives if their disabilities are properly managed. In general, the earlier treatment begins, the better chance children have of overcoming developmental disabilities or learning new ways to accomplish the tasks that challenge them.

There is no standard therapy that works for every individual with CP. Once the diagnosis is made, and the type of CP is determined, a team of healthcare professionals will work with a child and his or her parents to identify specific impairments and needs, and then develop an appropriate plan to tackle the core disabilities that affect the child's quality of life.

Chapter 24
Epilepsy Can Affect Learning

Epilepsy And Learning Disabilities

If one area of the brain is wired differently, it is not uncommon that other areas of the brain will be wired differently. The relationship between epilepsy and learning disabilities is but one example.

Epilepsy, also called seizure disorders, is characterized by recurrent seizures. It is associated with structural or biochemical brain abnormalities. It is estimated that 1 percent of the general population has epilepsy. This disorder occurs more commonly in boys than girls. About 40 percent of individuals with epilepsy between the ages of 4 and 15 have one or more additional neurological disorders. The most common ones are mental retardation, speech-language disabilities, and specific learning disabilities. In fact, learning disabilities are more prevalent in individuals with epilepsy (approaching 50%) than in the general population.

One of the most notable effects of cognitive functioning in children with epilepsy is memory impairment. This impairment can range from poor concentration and minor forgetfulness to gross clouding of consciousness and disorientation.

Epilepsy might impact learning in other ways. Daytime seizures can affect learning by reducing alertness and by interfering with short-term information storage and abstraction. Frequent and uncontrolled seizures impair learning new information due to the amount of

About This Chapter: Text under the heading "Epilepsy And Learning Disabilities" is excerpted from "Epilepsy And Learning Disabilities," © 2016 Learning Disabilities Association of America (LDA). Reprinted with permission; Text under the heading "Educational Implications" is excerpted from "Early Childhood Development, Teaching, and Learning: Epilepsy," Office of Head Start (OHS), Administration for Children and Families (ACF), U.S. Department of Health and Human Services (HHS), July 2014.

time that the individual is unaware of the environment. Night-time seizures can disrupt the consolidation of memory and affect language functions.

Cognitive impairments can also be a side effect of the various anticonvulsant medications used to treat epilepsy. Anticonvulsant medications have been associated with learning difficulty, behavior changes, and memory impairment. The drug most commonly implicated with altered behavior is phenobarbital, which can cause hyperactivity and memory impairment. Almost all anticonvulsant medications have some adverse effects on cognition, learning, and mood. Additional factors that are detrimental to learning include toxic levels of anticonvulsant drugs and the use of more than one antiepileptic medication. It is important when treating seizures in children with learning difficulties to carefully assess the medication used and the possible impact of this medication.

Characteristics Of Epilepsy

Although the symptoms listed below are not necessarily indicators of epilepsy, it is wise to consult a doctor if you or a member of your family experiences one or more of them:

- "blackouts" or periods of confused memory;
- episodes of staring or unexplained periods of unresponsiveness;
- involuntary movement of arms and legs;
- "fainting spells" with incontinence or followed by excessive fatigue; or
- odd sounds, distorted perceptions, episodic feelings of fear that cannot be explained.

Seizures can be generalized, meaning that all brain cells are involved. One type of generalized seizure consists of a convulsion with a complete loss of consciousness. Another type looks like a brief period of fixed staring.

Seizures are partial when those brain cells not working properly are limited to one part of the brain. Such partial seizures may cause periods of "automatic behavior" and altered consciousness. This is typified by purposeful-looking behavior, such as buttoning or unbuttoning a shirt. Such behavior, however, is unconscious, may be repetitive, and is usually not recalled.

(Source: "Early Childhood Development, Teaching, and Learning: Epilepsy," Office of Head Start (OHS), Administration for Children and Families (ACF), U.S. Department of Health and Human Services (HHS).)

Educational Implications

Seizures may interfere with the child's ability to learn. If the student has the type of seizure characterized by a brief period of fixed staring, he or she may be missing parts of what the teacher is saying. It is important that the teacher observe and document these episodes and report them promptly to parents and to school nurses.

Students with epilepsy or seizure disorders are eligible for special education and related services under the Individuals with Disabilities Education Act (IDEA). Epilepsy is classified as "other health impaired" and an Individualized Education Program (IEP) would be developed to specify appropriate services. Some students may have additional conditions such as learning disabilities along with the seizure disorders.

Depending on the type of seizure or how often they occur, some children may need additional assistance to help them keep up with classmates. Assistance can include adaptations in classroom instruction, first aid instruction on seizure management to the student's teachers, and counseling, all of which should be written in the IEP.

It is important that the teachers and school staff are informed about the child's condition, possible effects of medication, and what to do in case a seizure occurs at school. Most parents find that a friendly conversation with the teacher(s) at the beginning of the school year is the best way to handle the situation. Even if a child has seizures that are largely controlled by medication, it is still best to notify the school staff about the condition.

School personnel and the family should work together to monitor the effectiveness of medication as well as any side effects. If a child's physical or intellectual skills seem to change, it is important to tell the doctor. There may also be associated hearing or perception problems caused by the brain changes. Written observations of both the family and school staff will be helpful in discussions with the child's doctor.

Children and youth with epilepsy must also deal with the psychological and social aspects of the condition. These include public misperceptions and fear of seizures, uncertain occurrence, loss of self-control during the seizure episode, and compliance with medications. To help children feel more confident about themselves and accept their epilepsy, the school can assist by providing epilepsy education programs for staff and students, including information on seizure recognition and first aid.

Students can benefit the most when both the family and school are working together. There are many materials available for families and teachers so that they can understand how to work most effectively as a team.

Chapter 25
Autism And Communication

What Is Autism Spectrum Disorder?

Autism spectrum disorder (ASD) covers a set of developmental disabilities that can cause significant social, communication, and behavioral challenges. People with ASD process information in their brain differently than other people.

ASD affects people in different ways and can range from mild to severe. People with ASD share some symptoms, such as difficulties with social interaction, but there are differences in when the symptoms start, how severe they are, how many symptoms there are, and whether other problems are present.

The signs of ASD begin before the age of 3, although some children may show hints of future problems within the first year of life.

Who Is Affected By ASD?

ASD affects people of every race, ethnic group, and socioeconomic background, but it is five times more common among boys than among girls. The Centers for Disease Control and Prevention (CDC) estimates that about 1 out of every 88 children will be identified with ASD.

About This Chapter: This chapter includes text excerpted from "Autism Spectrum Disorder: Communication Problems In Children," National Institute on Deafness and Other Communication Disorders (NIDCD), March 21, 2016.

How Does Autism Spectrum Disorder Affect Communication?

The word "autism" has its origin in the Greek word "autos," which means "self." Children with ASD often are self-absorbed and seem to exist in a private world where they are unable to successfully communicate and interact with others. Children with ASD may have difficulty developing language skills and understanding what others say to them. They also may have difficulty communicating nonverbally, such as through hand gestures, eye contact, and facial expressions.

Not every child with ASD will have a language problem. A child's ability to communicate will vary, depending upon his or her intellectual and social development. Some children with ASD may be unable to speak. Others may have rich vocabularies and be able to talk about specific subjects in great detail. Most children with ASD have little or no problem pronouncing words. The majority, however, have difficulty using language effectively, especially when they talk to other people. Many have problems with the meaning and rhythm of words and sentences. They also may be unable to understand body language and the nuances of vocal tones.

Below are some patterns of language use and behaviors that are often found in children with ASD.

- **Repetitive or rigid language.** Often, children with ASD who can speak will say things that have no meaning or that seem out of context in conversations with others. For example, a child may count from one to five repeatedly. Or a child may repeat words he or she has heard over and over, a condition called **echolalia**. Immediate echolalia occurs when the child repeats words someone has just said. For example, the child may respond to a question by asking the same question. In delayed echolalia, the child will repeat words heard at an earlier time. The child may say "Do you want something to drink?" whenever he or she asks for a drink. Some children with ASD speak in a high-pitched or singsong voice or use robot-like speech. Other children may use stock phrases to start a conversation. For example, a child may say "My name is Tom," even when he talks with friends or family. Still others may repeat what they hear on television programs or commercials.

- **Narrow interests and exceptional abilities.** Some children may be able to deliver an in-depth monologue about a topic that holds their interest, even though they may not be able to carry on a two-way conversation about the same topic. Others have musical talents or an advanced ability to count and do math calculations. Approximately 10 percent of children with ASD show "savant" skills, or extremely high abilities in specific areas, such as calendar calculation, music, or math.

- **Uneven language development.** Many children with ASD develop some speech and language skills, but not to a normal level of ability, and their progress is usually uneven. For example, they may develop a strong vocabulary in a particular area of interest very quickly. Many children have good memories for information just heard or seen. Some children may be able to read words before 5 years of age, but they may not comprehend what they have read. They often do not respond to the speech of others and may not respond to their own names. As a result, these children sometimes are mistakenly thought to have a hearing problem.

- **Poor nonverbal conversation skills.** Children with ASD often are unable to use gestures—such as pointing to an object—to give meaning to their speech. They often avoid eye contact, which can make them seem rude, uninterested, or inattentive. Without meaningful gestures or the language to communicate, many children with ASD become frustrated in their attempts to make their feelings and needs known. They may act out their frustrations through vocal outbursts or other inappropriate behaviors.

How Are The Speech And Language Problems Of Autism Spectrum Disorder Treated?

If a doctor suspects a child has ASD or another developmental disability, he or she usually will refer the child to a variety of specialists, including a speech-language pathologist. This is a health professional trained to treat individuals with voice, speech, and language disorders. The speech-language pathologist will perform a comprehensive evaluation of the child's ability to communicate and design an appropriate treatment program. In addition, the pathologist might make a referral for audiological testing to make sure the child's hearing is normal.

Teaching children with ASD how to communicate is essential in helping them reach their full potential. There are many different approaches to improve communication skills. The best treatment program begins early, during the preschool years, and is tailored to the child's age and interests. It also will address both the child's behavior and communication skills and offer regular reinforcement of positive actions. Most children with ASD respond well to highly structured, specialized programs. Parents or primary caregivers, as well as other family members should be involved in the treatment program so it will become part of the child's daily life.

For some younger children, improving verbal communication is a realistic goal of treatment.

Parents and caregivers can increase a child's chance of reaching this goal by paying attention to his or her language development early on. Just as toddlers learn to crawl before they walk, children first develop pre-language skills before they begin to use words. These skills include using eye contact, gestures, body movements, and babbling and other vocalizations to help them communicate. Children who lack these skills may be evaluated and treated by a speech-language pathologist to prevent further developmental delays.

For slightly older children with ASD, basic communication training often emphasizes the functional use of language, such as learning to hold a conversation with another person, which includes staying on topic and taking turns speaking.

Some children with ASD may never develop verbal language skills. For them, the goal may be to acquire gestured communication, such as the use of sign language. For others, the goal may be to communicate by means of a symbol system in which pictures are used to convey thoughts. Symbol systems can range from picture boards or cards to sophisticated electronic devices that generate speech through the use of buttons that represent common items or actions.

What Research Is Being Conducted To Improve Communication In Children With Autism Spectrum Disorder?

The federal government's Combating Autism Act of 2006 brought attention to the need to expand research and improve coordination among all of the components of the National Institutes of Health (NIH) that fund research. These include the National Institute of Mental Health (NIMH), which is the principal institute for research at the NIH, along with the National Institute on Deafness and Other Communication Disorders (NIDCD), the *Eunice Kennedy Shriver* National Institute on Child Health and Human Development (NICHD), the National Institute of Environmental Health Sciences (NIEHS), and the National Institute of Neurological Disorders and Stroke (NINDS).

Together, these five institutes have established the Autism Centers of Excellence (ACE), a program of research centers and networks at universities across the country. Here, scientists study a broad range of topics, from basic science investigations that explore the molecular and genetic components of ASD to translational research studies that test new types of behavioral interventions. Some of these studies, which could be testing new treatments or interventions, might be of interest to parents of children with ASD.

The NIDCD supports additional research to improve the lives of people with ASD and their families. Recently, a group of NIDCD-funded researchers developed recommendations calling for a standardized approach to evaluating language skills. The new benchmarks will make it easier, and more accurate, to compare the effectiveness of different intervention strategies.

NIDCD-funded researchers in universities and organizations across the country also are looking at:

- How to better predict early in infancy if a child is at risk for ASD.

- Whether or not treatment interventions for at-risk infants can influence the development of speech perception and speech preferences.

- How infants with ASD "visually" scan their environment during their earliest social interactions and how this influences their development of language and communication skills.

- How genes and other potential factors predispose individuals to ASD.

Chapter 26

Down Syndrome And Learning Difficulties

Down syndrome is a chromosomal condition that is associated with intellectual disability, a characteristic facial appearance, and weak muscle tone (hypotonia) in infancy. All affected individuals experience cognitive delays, but the intellectual disability is usually mild to moderate.

People with Down syndrome may have a variety of birth defects. About half of all affected children are born with a heart defect. Digestive abnormalities, such as a blockage of the intestine, are less common.

Individuals with Down syndrome have an increased risk of developing several medical conditions. These include gastroesophageal reflux, which is a backflow of acidic stomach contents into the esophagus, and celiac disease, which is an intolerance of a wheat protein called gluten. About 15 percent of people with Down syndrome have an underactive thyroid gland (hypothyroidism). The thyroid gland is a butterfly-shaped organ in the lower neck that produces hormones. Individuals with Down syndrome also have an increased risk of hearing and vision problems. Additionally, a small percentage of children with Down syndrome develop cancer of blood-forming cells (leukemia).

People with Down syndrome often experience a gradual decline in thinking ability (cognition) as they age, usually starting around age 50. Down syndrome is also associated with an increased risk of developing Alzheimer disease, a brain disorder that results in a gradual loss of memory, judgment, and ability to function. Approximately half of adults with Down

About This Chapter: Text in this chapter begins with excerpts from "Down Syndrome," Genetics Home Reference (GHR), National Institutes of Health (NIH), June 2012. Reviewed December 2016; Text beginning with the heading "Common Physical Features" is excerpted from "Birth Defects: Facts About Down Syndrome," Division of Birth Defects and Developmental Disabilities (NCBDDD), Centers for Disease Control and Prevention (CDC), March 3, 2016.

Delayed development and behavioral problems are often reported in children with Down syndrome. Affected individuals' speech and language develop later and more slowly than in children without Down syndrome, and affected individuals' speech may be more difficult to understand. Behavioral issues can include attention problems, obsessive/compulsive behavior, and stubbornness or tantrums. A small percentage of people with Down syndrome are also diagnosed with developmental conditions called autism spectrum disorders, which affect communication and social interaction.

syndrome develop Alzheimer disease. Although Alzheimer disease is usually a disorder that occurs in older adults, people with Down syndrome usually develop this condition in their fifties or sixties.

Common Physical Features

Some common physical features of Down syndrome include:

- a flattened face, especially the bridge of the nose

- almond-shaped eyes that slant up

- a short neck

- small ears

- a tongue that tends to stick out of the mouth

- tiny white spots on the iris (colored part) of the eye

- small hands and feet

- a single line across the palm of the hand (palmar crease)

- small pinky fingers that sometimes curve toward the thumb

- poor muscle tone or loose joints

- shorter in height as children and adults

Even though people with Down syndrome might act and look similar, each person has different abilities. People with Down syndrome usually have an IQ (a measure of intelligence) in the mildly-to-moderately low range and are slower to speak than other children.

Types Of Down Syndrome

There are three types of Down syndrome. People often can't tell the difference between each type without looking at the chromosomes because the physical features and behaviors are similar.

- **Trisomy 21:** About 95 percent of people with Down syndrome have Trisomy 21. With this type of Down syndrome, each cell in the body has 3 separate copies of chromosome 21 instead of the usual 2 copies.

- **Translocation Down syndrome:** This type accounts for a small percentage of people with Down syndrome (about 3%). This occurs when an extra part or a whole extra chromosome 21 is present, but it is attached or "trans-located" to a different chromosome rather than being a separate chromosome 21.

- **Mosaic Down syndrome:** This type affects about 2 percent of the people with Down syndrome. Mosaic means mixture or combination. For children with mosaic Down syndrome, some of their cells have 3 copies of chromosome 21, but other cells have the typical two copies of chromosome 21. Children with mosaic Down syndrome may have the same features as other children with Down syndrome. However, they may have fewer features of the condition due to the presence of some (or many) cells with a typical number of chromosomes.

Diagnosis

There are two basic types of tests available to detect Down syndrome during pregnancy. Screening tests are one type and diagnostic tests are another type. A screening test can tell a woman and her healthcare provider whether her pregnancy has a lower or higher chance of having Down syndrome. So screening tests help decide whether a diagnostic test might be needed. Screening tests do not provide an absolute diagnosis, but they are safer for the mother and the baby. Diagnostic tests can typically detect whether or not a baby will have Down syndrome, but they can be more risky for the mother and baby. Neither screening nor diagnostic tests can predict the full impact of Down syndrome on a baby; no one can predict this.

Screening Tests

Screening tests often include a combination of a blood test, which measures the amount of various substances in the mother's blood (e.g., maternal serum alpha-fetoprotein (MS-AFP), Triple Screen, Quad-screen), and an ultrasound, which creates a picture of the baby. During an ultrasound, one of the things the technician looks at is the fluid behind the baby's neck. Extra fluid in this region could indicate a genetic problem. These screening tests can help determine the baby's risk of Down syndrome. Rarely, screening tests can give an abnormal result even when there is nothing wrong with the baby. Sometimes, the test results are normal and yet they miss a problem that does exist.

In recent years, noninvasive prenatal testing (NIPT) has become available to women who are at increased risk to have a baby with Down syndrome. NIPT is a blood test that examines DNA from the fetus in the mother's bloodstream. However, women who have a positive NIPT result should then have invasive diagnostic testing to confirm the result.

(Source: "Down Syndrome," Genetic and Rare Diseases Information Center (GARD), National Center for Advancing Translational Sciences (NCATS).)

Diagnostic Tests

Diagnostic tests are usually performed after a positive screening test in order to confirm a Down syndrome diagnosis. Types of diagnostic tests include:

- Chorionic villus sampling (CVS)—examines material from the placenta

- Amniocentesis—examines the amniotic fluid (the fluid from the sac surrounding the baby)

- Percutaneous umbilical blood sampling (PUBS)—examines blood from the umbilical cord

These tests look for changes in the chromosomes that would indicate a Down syndrome diagnosis.

Treatment

Down syndrome is a lifelong condition. Services early in life will often help babies and children with Down syndrome to improve their physical and intellectual abilities. Most of these services focus on helping children with Down syndrome develop to their full potential. These services include speech, occupational, and physical therapy, and they are typically offered through early intervention programs in each state. Children with Down syndrome may also need extra help or attention in school, although many children are included in regular classes.

Early intervention services, quality educational programs, a stimulating home environment, good healthcare, and positive support from family and friends can help people with Down syndrome develop to their full potential. The overall goal of treatment is to boost cognition by improving learning, memory, and speech. Other treatments depend on the specific health problems or complications present in each affected person.

(Source: "Down Syndrome," Genetic and Rare Diseases Information Center (GARD), National Center for Advancing Translational Sciences (NCATS).)

Chapter 27

Tourette Syndrome Associated With Learning Disabilities

Tourette Syndrome (TS) is a condition of the nervous system. TS causes people to have "tics."

Tics are sudden twitches, movements, or sounds that people do repeatedly. People who have tics cannot stop their body from doing these things. For example, a person might keep blinking over and over again. Or, a person might make a grunting sound unwillingly.

Having tics is a little bit like having hiccups. Even though you might not want to hiccup, your body does it anyway. Sometimes people can stop themselves from doing a certain tic for awhile, but it's hard. Eventually, the person has to do the tic.

Types of Tics

There are two types of tics—motor and vocal:

- **Motor Tics:** Motor tics are movements of the body. Examples of motor tics include blinking, shrugging the shoulders, or jerking an arm.

- **Vocal Tics:** Vocal tics are sounds that a person makes with his or her voice. Examples of vocal tics include humming, clearing the throat, or yelling out a word or phrase.

Tics can be either simple or complex:

- **Simple Tics:** Simple tics involve just a few parts of the body. Examples of simple tics include squinting the eyes or sniffing.

About This Chapter: This chapter includes text excerpted from "Tourette Syndrome (TS)," National Center on Birth Defects and Developmental Disabilities (NCBDDD), Centers for Disease Control and Prevention (CDC), November 30, 2015.

- **Complex Tics:** Complex tics usually involve several different parts of the body and can have a pattern. An example of a complex tic is bobbing the head while jerking an arm, and then jumping up.

Symptoms

The main symptoms of TS are tics. Symptoms usually begin when a child is 5 to 10 years of age. The first symptoms often are motor tics that occur in the head and neck area. Tics usually are worse during times that are stressful or exciting. They tend to improve when a person is calm or focused on an activity.

The types of tics and how often a person has tics changes a lot over time. Even though the symptoms might appear, disappear, and reappear, these conditions are considered chronic.

In most cases, tics decrease during adolescence and early adulthood, and sometimes disappear entirely. However, many people with TS experience tics into adulthood and, in some cases, tics can become worse during adulthood.

Although the media often portray people with TS as involuntarily shouting out swear words (called coprolalia) or constantly repeating the words of other people (called echolalia), these symptoms are rare, and are not required for a diagnosis of TS.

Diagnosis

The American Psychiatric Association's *Diagnostic and Statistical Manual of Mental Disorders, Fifth Edition (DSM-5)* is used by health professionals to help diagnose tic disorders.

Three tic disorders are included in the DSM-5:

- Tourette's disorder (also called Tourette syndrome (TS))

- Persistent (also called chronic) motor or vocal tic disorder

- Provisional tic disorder

The tic disorders differ from each other in terms of the type of tic present (motor or vocal, or a combination of both), and how long the symptoms have lasted. People with TS have both motor and vocal tics, and have had tic symptoms for at least 1 year. People with persistent motor or vocal tic disorders have either motor or vocal tics, and have had tic symptoms for at least 1 year. People with provisional tic disorders can have motor or vocal tics, or both, but have had their symptoms less than 1 year.

Please note that they are presented for your information only and should not be used for self-diagnosis. If you are concerned about any of the symptoms listed, you should consult a trained healthcare provider with experience in diagnosing and treating tic disorders.

Tourette Syndrome

For a person to be diagnosed with TS, he or she must:

- Have two or more motor tics (for example, blinking or shrugging the shoulders) and at least one vocal tic (for example, humming, clearing the throat, or yelling out a word or phrase), although they might not always happen at the same time.

- Have had tics for at least a year. The tics can occur many times a day (usually in bouts) nearly every day, or off and on.

- Have tics that begin before he or she is 18 years of age.

- Have symptoms that are not due to taking medicine or other drugs or due to having another medical condition (for example, seizures, Huntington disease, or postviral encephalitis).

Persistent (Chronic) Motor Or Vocal Tic Disorder

For a person to be diagnosed with a persistent tic disorder, he or she must:

- Have one or more motor tics (for example, blinking or shrugging the shoulders) or vocal tics (for example, humming, clearing the throat, or yelling out a word or phrase), but not both.

- Have tics that occur many times a day nearly every day or on and off throughout a period of more than a year.

- Have tics that start before he or she is 18 years of age.

- Have symptoms that are not due to taking medicine or other drugs, or due to having a medical condition that can cause tics (for example, seizures, Huntington disease, or postviral encephalitis).

- Not have been diagnosed with TS.

Provisional Tic Disorder

For a person to be diagnosed with this disorder, he or she must:

- Have one or more motor tics (for example, blinking or shrugging the shoulders) or vocal tics (for example, humming, clearing the throat, or yelling out a word or phrase).

- Have been present for no longer than 12 months in a row.

- Have tics that start before he or she is 18 years of age.

- Have symptoms that are not due to taking medicine or other drugs, or due to having a medical condition that can cause tics (for example, Huntington disease or postviral encephalitis).

- Not have been diagnosed with TS or persistent motor or vocal tic disorder.

Treatments

Although there is no cure for TS, there are treatments to help manage the tics caused by TS. Many people with TS have tics that do not get in the way of their living their daily life and, therefore, do not need any treatment. However, medication and behavioral treatments are available if tics cause pain or injury; interfere with school, work, or social life; or cause stress. A promising new behavioral treatment is the Comprehensive Behavioral Intervention for Tics (CBIT)

Educating the community (for example, peers, educators, and coworkers) about TS can increase understanding of the symptoms, reduce teasing, and decrease stress for people living with TS. People with TS cannot help having tics, and are not being disruptive on purpose. When others understand these facts, people with TS might receive more support, which might, in turn, help lessen some tic symptoms.

It is common for people with TS to have co-occurring conditions, particularly attention deficit hyperactivity disorder (ADHD) and obsessive compulsive disorder (OCD). People with additional conditions will require different treatments based on the symptoms. Sometimes treating these other conditions can help reduce tics. To develop the best treatment plan, people with tics, parents, and healthcare providers should work closely with one another, and with everyone involved in treatment and support—which may include teachers, childcare providers, coaches, therapists, and other family members. Taking advantage of all the resources available will help guide success.

Medications

Medications can be used to reduce severe or disruptive tics that might have led to problems in the past with family and friends, other students, or coworkers. Medications also can be used to reduce symptoms of related conditions, such as ADHD or OCD.

Medications do not eliminate tics completely. However, they can help some people with TS in their everyday life. There is no one medication that is best for all people. Most medications prescribed for TS have not been approved by the U.S. Food and Drug Administration (FDA) for treating tics.

Medications affect each person differently. One person might do well with one medication, but not another. When deciding the best treatment, a doctor might try different medications and doses, and it may take time to find the treatment plan that works best. The doctor will want to find the medication and dose that have the best results and the fewest side effects. Doctors often start with small doses and slowly increase as needed.

> As with all medications, those used to treat tics can have side effects. Side effects can include weight gain, stiff muscles, tiredness, restlessness, and social withdrawal. The side effects need to be considered carefully when deciding whether or not to use any medication to treat tics. In some cases, the side effects can be worse than the tics.
>
> Even though medications often are used to treat the symptoms of TS, they might not be helpful for everyone. Two common reasons for not using medications to treat TS are unpleasant side effects and failure of the medications to work as well as expected.

Behavioral Therapy

Behavioral therapy is a treatment that teaches people with TS ways to manage their tics. Behavioral therapy is not a cure for tics. However, it can help reduce the number of tics, the severity of tics, the impact of tics, or a combination of all of these.

Habit Reversal

Habit reversal is one of the most studied behavioral interventions for people with tics. It has two main parts: awareness training and competing response training. In the awareness training part, people identify each tic out loud. In the competing response part, people learn to do a new behavior that cannot happen at the same time as the tic. For example, if the person with TS has a tic that involves head rubbing, a new behavior might be for that person to place his or her hands on his or her knees, or to cross his or her arms so that the head rubbing cannot take place.

Comprehensive Behavioral Intervention For Tics

CBIT is a new, evidence-based type of behavioral therapy for TS and chronic tic disorders. CBIT includes habit reversal in addition to other strategies, including education about tics and relaxation techniques. CBIT has been shown to be effective at reducing tic symptoms and tic-related impairment among children and adults.

In CBIT, a therapist will work with a child (and his or her parents) or an adult with TS to better understand the types of tics the person is having and to understand the situations in which the tics are at their worst. Changes to the surroundings may be made, if possible, and the person with TS will also learn to do a new behavior instead of the tic (habit reversal). For example, if a child with TS often has a certain tic during math class, the math teacher can be educated about TS, and perhaps the child's seat can be changed so that the tics are not as visible. In addition, the child also can work with a psychologist to learn habit reversal techniques. This helps to decrease how often the tic occurs by doing a new behavior (like putting his or her hands on his or her knees when an urge to perform the tic happens). CBIT skills can be learned with practice, with the help of an experienced therapist, and with the support and encouragement of those close to the person with TS.

In recent years, more health professionals have recognized that behavioral therapy can be very effective in managing the symptoms of TS.

Parent Training

Children with TS and related conditions and their families also can benefit from parent training, which has been shown to be successful among children with both TS and other disruptive behaviors. Parent training also has been shown to be helpful for children with ADHD. Parent training helps parents better understand their child's behavioral issues and learn parenting skills specific to these problems. The training might include learning about the effective use of positive reinforcement and discipline that is effective with their particular child.

Other Concerns And Conditions

TS often occurs with other related conditions (also called co-occurring conditions). These conditions can include ADHD, OCD, and other behavioral or conduct problems. People with TS and related conditions can be at higher risk for learning, behavioral, and social problems.

The symptoms of other disorders can complicate the diagnosis and treatment of TS and create extra challenges for people with TS and their families, educators, and health professionals.

Findings from a national Centers for Disease Control and Prevention (CDC) study indicated that 86% of children who had been diagnosed with TS also had been diagnosed with at least one additional mental health, behavioral, or developmental condition based on parent report.

Among children with TS:

- 63% had ADHD

- 26% had behavioral problems, such as oppositional defiant disorder (ODD) or conduct disorder (CD)

- 49% had anxiety problems

- 25% had depression

- 35% had an autism spectrum disorder

- 47% had a learning disability

- 29% had a speech or language problem

- 30% had a developmental delay

- 12% had an intellectual disability

Because co-occurring conditions are so common among people with TS, it is important for doctors to assess every child with TS for other conditions and problems.

Risk Factors And Causes

Scientists are studying the causes of and risk factors for TS in an effort to understand it better, and to find better ways to manage TS and to reduce the chances of a person having TS. The causes of TS and other tic disorders are not well understood.

Although the risk factors for and causes of TS are unknown, current research shows that genes play an important role:

- Genetic studies have indicated that TS is inherited as a dominant gene, with about a 50% chance of parents passing the gene on to their children.

- Boys with the gene(s) are three to four times more likely than girls to display symptoms of TS.

- TS can be triggered by abnormal metabolism (breakdown) of a chemical in the brain called dopamine.

Some research has shown that TS is a genetically complex disorder that likely occurs as a result of the effects of multiple genes interacting with other factors in the environment. Scientists are studying other possible causes and environmental risk factors that might contribute to TS. Some studies have shown that the following factors might be associated with TS, but additional research is needed to better understand these associations:

- Mother drinking alcohol or smoking during pregnancy.

- Complications during birth.

- Low birthweight.

- Infection. Researchers are investigating whether certain children are more likely to develop tics following a group A ß-hemolytic streptococcal ("strep") infection. This is referred to as Pediatric Autoimmune Neuropsychiatric Disorders Associated with Streptococcal (PANDAS) infections.

Who Is Affected?

In the United States, 1 of every 360 children 6 through 17 years of age have been diagnosed with TS. TS can affect people of all racial and ethnic groups. Boys are affected three to five times more often than girls.

What Is The Best Educational Setting For Children With Tourette Syndrome?

Although students with TS often function well in the regular classroom, ADHD, learning disabilities, obsessive compulsive symptoms, and frequent tics can greatly interfere with academic performance or social adjustment. After a comprehensive assessment, students should be placed in an educational setting that meets their individual needs. Students may require tutoring, smaller or special classes, and in some cases special schools.

All students with TS need a tolerant and compassionate setting that both encourages them to work to their full potential and is flexible enough to accommodate their special needs. This setting may include a private study area, exams outside the regular classroom, or even oral exams when the child's symptoms interfere with his or her ability to write. Untimed testing reduces stress for students with TS.

(Source: "Tourette Syndrome Fact Sheet," National Institute of Neurological Disorders and Stroke (NINDS).)

Chapter 28

Abusive Head Trauma (Shaken Baby Syndrome)

Abusive head trauma (AHT), also called shaken baby syndrome (or SBS), goes by many other names, including inflicted traumatic brain injury and shaken impact syndrome. All of these names mean the same thing: an injury to a child's brain as a result of child abuse.

Abusive head trauma (AHT) can be caused by direct blows to the head, dropping or throwing a child, or shaking a child. Head trauma is the leading cause of death in child abuse cases in the United States. Because the anatomy of infants puts them at particular risk for injury from this kind of action, the majority of victims are infants younger than 1 year old.

AHT can happen in children up to 5 years old, and the average age of victims is between 3 and 8 months. However, the highest rate of cases occur among infants just 6 to 8 weeks old, which is when babies tend to cry the most.

How These Injuries Happen

Abusive head trauma results from injuries caused by someone (most often a parent or other caregiver) vigorously shaking a child or striking the child's head against a surface. In many cases, the caregiver cannot get the baby to stop crying and, out of frustration or anger, will shake the baby. Unfortunately, the shaking may have the desired effect: Although at first the baby cries more, he or she may stop crying as the brain is damaged.

Children with special needs, multiple siblings, or conditions like colic or gastroesophageal reflux disease (GERD) have an increased risk of AHT. Boys are more likely to be victims

---

About This Chapter: Text in this chapter is excerpted from "Abusive Head Trauma (Shaken Baby Syndrome)," © 1995–2016. The Nemours Foundation/KidsHealth®. Reprinted with permission.

of AHT than girls, and children of families who live at or below the poverty level are at an increased risk for these injuries and other types of child abuse.

The perpetrators in about 70 percent of cases are males—usually either the baby's father or the mother's boyfriend, often someone in his early twenties. But anyone has the potential to shake a baby if he or she isn't able to handle stressful situations well, has poor impulse control, or has a tendency toward aggressive behavior. Substance abuse often plays a role in AHT.

When someone forcefully shakes a baby, the child's head rotates uncontrollably. This is because infants' neck muscles aren't well developed and provide little support for their heads. This violent movement pitches the infant's brain back and forth within the skull, sometimes rupturing blood vessels and nerves throughout the brain and tearing the brain tissue. The brain may strike the inside of the skull, causing bruising and bleeding to the brain.

The damage can be even greater when a shaking episode ends with an impact (hitting a wall or a crib mattress, for example) because the forces of acceleration and deceleration associated with an impact are so strong. After the shaking, swelling in the brain can cause enormous pressure within the skull, compressing blood vessels and increasing overall injury to the brain's delicate structure.

Normal interaction with a child, like bouncing the baby on a knee or tossing the baby up in the air, will **not** cause these injuries. But it's important to **never** shake a baby under **any** circumstances.

What Are The Effects?

AHT often causes irreversible damage, and about 1 out of every 4 cases results in the child's death.

Children who survive may have:

- partial or total blindness

- hearing loss

- seizures

- developmental delays

- impaired intellect

- speech and learning difficulties

- problems with memory and attention

- severe mental retardation

- cerebral palsy

Even in milder cases, in which babies look normal immediately after the shaking, they may eventually develop one or more of these problems. Sometimes the first sign of a problem isn't noticed until the child enters the school system and exhibits behavioral problems or learning difficulties. But by that time, it's more difficult to link these problems to a shaking incident from several years before.

Signs And Symptoms

In any abusive head trauma case, the duration and force of the shaking, the number of episodes, and whether impact is involved all affect the severity of the child's injuries. In the most violent cases, children may arrive at the emergency room unconscious, suffering seizures, or in shock. But in many cases, infants may *never* be brought to medical attention if they don't exhibit such severe symptoms.

In less severe cases, a child who has been shaken may experience:

- lethargy

- irritability

- vomiting

- poor sucking or swallowing

- decreased appetite

- lack of smiling or vocalizing

- rigidity

- seizures

- difficulty breathing

- blue color due to lack of oxygen

- altered consciousness

- unequal pupil size

- an inability to lift the head

- an inability to focus the eyes or track movement

Diagnosis

Many cases of AHT are brought in for medical care as "silent injuries." In other words, parents or caregivers don't often provide a history that the child has had abusive head trauma or a shaking injury, so doctors don't know to look for subtle or physical signs. This can sometimes result in children having injuries that aren't identified in the medical system.

In many cases, babies who don't have severe symptoms may *never* be brought to a doctor. Many of the less severe symptoms such as vomiting or irritability may resolve and can have many non-abuse-related causes.

Unfortunately, unless a doctor has reason to suspect child abuse, mild cases (in which the infant seems lethargic, fussy, or perhaps isn't feeding well) are often misdiagnosed as a viral illness or colic. Without a suspicion of child abuse and any resulting intervention with the parents or caregivers, these children may be shaken again, worsening any brain injury or damage.

If shaken baby syndrome *is* suspected, doctors may look for:

- hemorrhages in the retinas of the eyes

- skull fractures

- swelling of the brain

- subdural hematomas (blood collections pressing on the surface of the brain)

- rib and long bone (bones in the arms and legs) fractures

- bruises around the head, neck, or chest

The Child's Development And Education

What makes AHT so devastating is that it often involves a total brain injury. For example, a child whose vision is severely impaired won't be able to learn through observation, which decreases the child's overall ability to learn.

The development of language, vision, balance, and motor coordination, all of which occur to varying degrees after birth, are particularly likely to be affected in any child who has AHT. Such impairment can require intensive physical and occupational therapy to help the child acquire skills that would have developed normally had the brain injury not occurred.

Before age 3, a child can receive free speech or physical therapy through state-run early intervention programs. Federal law requires that each state provide these services for children who have developmental disabilities as a result of being abused. After a child turns 3, it's the school district's responsibility to provide any needed additional special educational services.

As kids get older, they may require special education and continued therapy to help with language development and daily living skills, like dressing.

Preventing Abusive Head Trauma

Abusive head trauma is *100 percent preventable*. A key aspect of prevention is increasing awareness of the potential dangers of shaking.

Finding ways to alleviate the parent or caregiver's stress at the critical moments when a baby is crying can significantly reduce the risk to a child. Some hospital-based programs have helped new parents identify and prevent shaking injuries and understand how to respond when infants cry.

All Babies Cry is a national program that promotes healthy parenting behavior through practical demonstrations of infant soothing and ways to manage the stress of parenting. The program is divided into four parts: 1. What's normal about crying? 2. Comforting your baby. 3. Self-care tips for parents. 4. Colic and how to cope.

The National Center on Shaken Baby Syndrome offers a prevention program, the **Period of Purple Crying**, which can help parents and other caregivers understand crying in healthy infants and how to handle it.

Another method that can help is the **"five S's" approach**, which stands for:

1. Shushing (by using "white noise" or rhythmic sounds that mimic the constant whir of noise in the womb. Vacuum cleaners, hair dryers, clothes dryers, a running tub, or a white noise machine can all create this effect.)

2. Side/stomach positioning (placing the baby on the left side—to help with digestion—or on the belly while holding him or her. Babies should always be placed on their backs to sleep.)

3. Sucking (letting the baby breastfeed or bottle-feed, or giving the baby a pacifier or finger to suck on).

4. Swaddling (wrapping the baby in a blanket like a "burrrito" to help him or her feel more secure. Hips and knees should be slightly bent and turned out).

5. Swinging gently (rocking in a chair, using an infant swing, or taking a car ride to help duplicate the constant motion the baby felt in the womb).

If a baby in your care won't stop crying, you can also try the following:

- Make sure the baby's basic needs are met (for example, he or she isn't hungry and doesn't need to be changed).

- Check for signs of illness, like fever or swollen gums.

- Rock or walk with the baby.

- Sing or talk to the baby.

- Offer the baby a pacifier or a noisy toy.

- Take the baby for a ride in a stroller or strapped into a child safety seat in the car.

- Hold the baby close against your body and breathe calmly and slowly.

- Give the baby a warm bath.

- Pat or rub the baby's back.

- Call a friend or relative for support or to take care of the baby while you take a break.

- If nothing else works, put the baby on his or her back in the crib, close the door, and check on the baby in 10 minutes.

- Call your doctor if nothing seems to be helping your infant, in case there is a medical reason for the fussiness.

To prevent potential AHT, parents and caregivers of infants need to learn how to respond to their own stress. It's important to tell *anyone* caring for a baby to never shake him or her. Talk about the dangers of shaking and how it can be prevented.

Chapter 29
XYY Syndrome

47,XYY syndrome is characterized by an extra copy of the Y chromosome in each of a male's cells. Although males with this condition may be taller than average, this chromosomal change typically causes no unusual physical features. Most males with 47,XYY syndrome have normal sexual development and are able to father children.

47,XYY syndrome is associated with an increased risk of learning disabilities and delayed development of speech and language skills. Delayed development of motor skills (such as sitting and walking), weak muscle tone (hypotonia), hand tremors or other involuntary movements (motor tics), and behavioral and emotional difficulties are also possible. These characteristics vary widely among affected boys and men.

A small percentage of males with 47,XYY syndrome are diagnosed with autistic spectrum disorders, which are developmental conditions that affect communication and social interaction.

Frequency

This condition occurs in about 1 in 1,000 newborn boys. Five to 10 boys with 47,XYY syndrome are born in the United States each day.

Genetic Changes

People normally have 46 chromosomes in each cell. Two of the 46 chromosomes, known as X and Y, are called sex chromosomes because they help determine whether a person will

About This Chapter: This chapter includes text excerpted from "47,XYY Syndrome," Genetics Home Reference (GHR), National Institutes of Health (NIH), January 2009. Reviewed December 2016.

XYY Syndrome

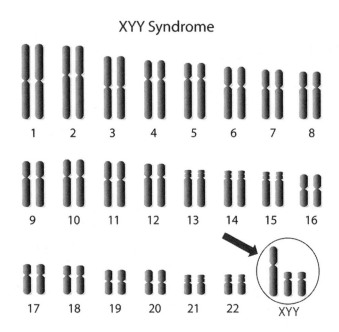

Figure 29.1. XYY Syndrome Karyotype

develop male or female sex characteristics. Females typically have two X chromosomes (46,XX), and males have one X chromosome and one Y chromosome (46,XY).

47,XYY syndrome is caused by the presence of an extra copy of the Y chromosome in each of a male's cells. As a result of the extra Y chromosome, each cell has a total of 47 chromosomes instead of the usual 46. It is unclear why an extra copy of the Y chromosome is associated with tall stature, learning problems, and other features in some boys and men.

Some males with 47,XYY syndrome have an extra Y chromosome in only some of their cells. This phenomenon is called 46,XY/47,XYY mosaicism.

Inheritance Pattern

Most cases of 47,XYY syndrome are not inherited. The chromosomal change usually occurs as a random event during the formation of sperm cells. An error in cell division called nondisjunction can result in sperm cells with an extra copy of the Y chromosome. If one of these atypical reproductive cells contributes to the genetic makeup of a child, the child will have an extra Y chromosome in each of the body's cells.

46,XY/47,XYY mosaicism is also not inherited. It occurs as a random event during cell division in early embryonic development. As a result, some of an affected person's cells have one X chromosome and one Y chromosome (46,XY), and other cells have one X chromosome and two Y chromosomes (47,XYY).

Other Names For This Condition

- Jacob syndrome
- XYY Karyotype
- 47,XYY Syndrome
- YY syndrome

Chapter 30

Triple X Syndrome

Triple X syndrome, also called trisomy X or 47,XXX, is characterized by the presence of an additional X chromosome in each of a female's cells. Although females with this condition may be taller than average, this chromosomal change typically causes no unusual physical features. Most females with triple X syndrome have normal sexual development and are able to conceive children.

> Triple X syndrome is associated with an increased risk of learning disabilities and delayed development of speech and language skills. Delayed development of motor skills (such as sitting and walking), weak muscle tone (hypotonia), and behavioral and emotional difficulties are also possible, but these characteristics vary widely among affected girls and women. Seizures or kidney abnormalities occur in about 10 percent of affected females.

Frequency

This condition occurs in about 1 in 1,000 newborn girls. Five to 10 girls with triple X syndrome are born in the United States each day.

Genetic Changes

People normally have 46 chromosomes in each cell. Two of the 46 chromosomes, known as X and Y, are called sex chromosomes because they help determine whether a person will

About This Chapter: Text in this chapter begins with excerpts from "Triple X Syndrome," Genetics Home Reference (GHR), National Institutes of Health (NIH), June 2014; Text beginning with the heading "Symptoms" is excerpted from "47 XXX Syndrome," Genetic and Rare Diseases Information Center (GARD), National Center for Advancing Translational Sciences (NCATS), December 2016.

Triple X Syndrome

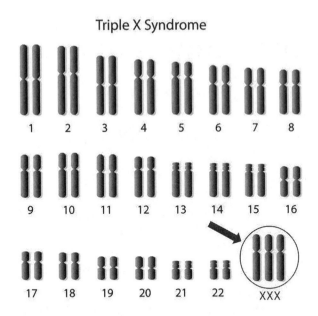

Figure 30.1. Triple X Syndrome Karyotype

develop male or female sex characteristics. Females typically have two X chromosomes (46,XX), and males have one X chromosome and one Y chromosome (46,XY).

Triple X syndrome results from an extra copy of the X chromosome in each of a female's cells. As a result of the extra X chromosome, each cell has a total of 47 chromosomes (47,XXX) instead of the usual 46. An extra copy of the X chromosome is associated with tall stature, learning problems, and other features in some girls and women.

Some females with triple X syndrome have an extra X chromosome in only some of their cells. This phenomenon is called 46,XX/47,XXX mosaicism.

Symptoms

Many women with 47,XXX syndrome have no symptoms or only mild symptoms. In other cases, symptoms may be more pronounced. Females with 47,XXX syndrome may be taller than average, but the condition usually does not cause unusual physical features. Minor physical findings can be present in some individuals and may include epicanthal folds, hypertelorism (widely spaced eyes), upslanting palpebral fissures, clinodactyly, overlapping digits (fingers or toes), pes planus (flat foot), and pectus excavatum.

Signs And Symptoms

- Abnormality of chromosome segregation
- Clinodactyly of the 5th finger
- Cognitive impairment
- Epicanthus
- Muscular hypotonia
- Tall stature
- Abnormality of the hip bone
- Attention deficit hyperactivity disorder
- Hypertelorism
- Joint hypermobility
- Multicystic kidney dysplasia
- Pectus excavatum
- Renal hypoplasia/aplasia
- Secondary amenorrhea
- Seizures
- Tremor
- Upslanted palpebral fissure

Inheritance

Most cases of 47,XXX syndrome are not inherited. The chromosomal change usually occurs as a random event during the formation of reproductive cells (eggs and sperm). An error in cell division called nondisjunction can result in reproductive cells with an abnormal number of chromosomes.

Diagnosis

47,XXX syndrome may first be suspected based on the presence of certain developmental, behavioral or learning disabilities in an individual. The diagnosis can be confirmed with chromosomal analysis (karyotyping), which can be performed on a blood sample. This test would reveal the presence of an extra X chromosome in body cells. 47,XXX syndrome may also be identified before birth (prenatally), based on chromosomal analysis performed on a sample taken during an amniocentesis or by a chorionic villus sampling (CVS) procedure. However, in these cases, confirmation testing with a test called FISH (fluorescent *in situ* hybridization), which gives more details of the chromosomes, is recommended in order to evaluate the fetus for mosaicism (when only some of the cells have the extra X chromosome).

Treatment

There is no cure for 47,XXX syndrome, and there is no way to remove the extra X chromosome that is present in an affected individual's cells. Management of the condition varies and depends on several factors including the age at diagnosis, the specific symptoms that are present, and the overall severity of the disorder in the affected individual. Recommendations include:

- early intervention services for infants and children that are diagnosed with the condition
- periodic screenings throughout childhood
- educational assistance
- supportive environment and counseling
- assistance and support in daily functioning

It is also recommended that infants and children with 47,XXX syndrome receive kidney and heart evaluations to detect possible abnormalities. Adolescent and adult women who have late periods, menstrual abnormalities, or fertility issues should be evaluated for primary ovarian failure (POF). Additional treatment for this disorder depends on the specific signs and symptoms present in the affected individual.

Other Names

- 47 XXX syndrome
- Triple X female
- XXX syndrome
- Triple-X chromosome syndrome
- Triplo X syndrome

Chapter 31

Klinefelter Syndrome

What Is Klinefelter Syndrome (KS)?

The term "Klinefelter syndrome," or KS, describes a set of features that can occur in a male who is born with an extra X chromosome in his cells. It is named after Dr. Henry Klinefelter, who identified the condition in the 1940s.

Usually, every cell in a male's body, except sperm and red blood cells, contains 46 chromosomes. The 45th and 46th chromosomes—the X and Y chromosomes—are sometimes called "sex chromosomes" because they determine a person's sex. Normally, males have one X and one Y chromosome, making them XY. Males with KS have an extra X chromosome, making them XXY.

KS is sometimes called "47,XXY" (47 refers to total chromosomes) or the "XXY condition." Those with KS are sometimes called "XXY males."

Some males with KS may have both XY cells and XXY cells in their bodies. This is called "mosaic." Mosaic males may have fewer symptoms of KS depending on the number of XY cells they have in their bodies and where these cells are located. For example, males who have normal XY cells in their testes may be fertile.

In very rare cases, males might have two or more extra X chromosomes in their cells, for instance XXXY or XXXXY, or an extra Y, such as XXYY. This is called poly-X Klinefelter syndrome, and it causes more severe symptoms.

About This Chapter: This chapter includes text excerpted from "Klinefelter Syndrome (KS)," *Eunice Kennedy Shriver* National Institute of Child Health and Human Development (NICHD), December 6, 2012. Reviewed December 2016.

What Causes Klinefelter Syndrome?

The extra chromosome results from a random error that occurs when a sperm or egg is formed; this error causes an extra X cell to be included each time the cell divides to form new cells. In very rare cases, more than one extra X or an extra Y is included.

What Are Common Symptoms Of Klinefelter Syndrome?

Because XXY males do not really appear different from other males and because they may not have any or have mild symptoms, XXY males often don't know they have KS.

In other cases, males with KS may have mild or severe symptoms. Whether or not a male with KS has visible symptoms depends on many factors, including how much testosterone his body makes, if he is mosaic (with both XY and XXY cells), and his age when the condition is diagnosed and treated.

KS symptoms fall into these main categories:

- Physical symptoms

- Language and learning symptoms

- Social and behavioral symptoms

- Symptoms of poly-X KS

Physical Symptoms

Many physical symptoms of KS result from low testosterone levels in the body. The degree of symptoms differs based on the amount of testosterone needed for a specific age or developmental stage and the amount of testosterone the body makes or has available.

During the first few years of life, when the need for testosterone is low, most XXY males do not show any obvious differences from typical male infants and young boys. Some may have slightly weaker muscles, meaning they might sit up, crawl, and walk slightly later than average. For example, on average, baby boys with KS do not start walking until age 18 months.

After age 5 years, when compared to typically developing boys, boys with KS may be slightly:

- taller

- fatter around the belly

- clumsier

- slower in developing motor skills, coordination, speed, and muscle strength

Puberty for boys with KS usually starts normally. But because their bodies make less testosterone than non-KS boys, their pubertal development may be disrupted or slow. In addition to being tall, KS boys may have:

- smaller testes and penis

- breast growth (about one-third of teens with KS have breast growth)

- less facial and body hair

- reduced muscle tone

- narrower shoulders and wider hips

- weaker bones, greater risk for bone fractures

- decreased sexual interest

- lower energy

- reduced sperm production

An adult male with KS may have these features:

- Infertility: Nearly all men with KS are unable to father a biologically-related child without help from a fertility specialist.

- Small testes, with the possibility of testes shrinking slightly after the teen years

- Lower testosterone levels, which lead to less muscle, hair, and sexual interest and function

- Breasts or breast growth (called gynecomastia)

In some cases, breast growth can be permanent, and about 10 percent of XXY males need breast-reduction surgery.

Language And Learning Symptoms

Most males with KS have normal intelligence quotients (IQs) and successfully complete education at all levels. (IQ is a frequently used intelligence measure, but does not include emotional, creative, or other types of intelligence.) Between 25 percent and 85 percent of all males with KS have some kind of learning or language-related problem, which makes it more likely that they will need some extra help in school. Without this help or intervention, KS males might fall behind their classmates as schoolwork becomes harder.

KS males may experience some of the following learning and language-related challenges:

- a delay in learning to talk

- trouble using language to express their thoughts and needs

- trouble processing what they hear

- reading difficulties

By adulthood, most males with KS learn to speak and converse normally, although they may have a harder time doing work that involves extensive reading and writing.

Social And Behavioral Symptoms

Many of the social and behavioral symptoms in KS may result from the language and learning difficulties. For instance, boys with KS who have language difficulties might hold back socially and could use help building social relationships.

Boys with KS, compared to typically developing boys, tend to be:

- quieter

- less assertive or self-confident

- more anxious or restless

- less physically active

- more helpful and eager to please

- more obedient or more ready to follow directions

In the teenage years, boys with KS may feel their differences more strongly. As a result, these teen boys are at higher risk of depression, substance abuse, and behavioral disorders. Some teens might withdraw, feel sad, or act out their frustration and anger.

As adults, most men with KS have lives similar to those of men without KS. They successfully complete high school, college, and other levels of education. They have successful and meaningful careers and professions. They have friends and families.

Symptoms Of Poly-X KS

Males with poly-X Klinefelter syndrome have more than one extra X chromosome, so their symptoms might be more pronounced than in males with KS. In childhood, they may also have seizures, crossed eyes, constipation, and recurrent ear infections. Poly-KS males might also show slight differences in other physical features.

Some common additional symptoms for several poly-X Klinefelter syndromes are listed below.

48,XXYY

- Long legs

- Little body hair

- Lower IQ, average of 60 to 80 (normal IQ is 90 to 110)

- Leg ulcers and other vascular disease symptoms

- Extreme shyness, but also sometimes aggression and impulsiveness

48,XXXY (or tetrasomy)

- Eyes set further apart

- Flat nose bridge

- Arm bones connected to each other in an unusual way

- Short

- Fifth (smallest) fingers curve inward (clinodactyly)

- Lower IQ, average 40 to 60

- Immature behavior

49,XXXXY (or pentasomy)

- Low IQ, usually between 20 and 60

- Small head

- Short

- Upward-slanted eyes

- Heart defects, such as when the chambers do not form properly

- High feet arches

- Shy, but friendly

- Difficulty with changing routines

What Are The Treatments For Symptoms In Klinefelter Syndrome?

It's important to remember that because symptoms can be mild, many males with KS are never diagnosed or treated.

The earlier in life that KS symptoms are recognized and treated, the more likely it is that the symptoms can be reduced or eliminated. It is especially helpful to begin treatment by early puberty. Puberty is a time of rapid physical and psychological change, and treatment can successfully limit symptoms. However, treatment can bring benefits at any age.

The type of treatment needed depends on the type of symptoms being treated.

- Treating physical symptoms
- Treating language and learning symptoms
- Treating social and behavioral symptoms

Treating Physical Symptoms

Treatment For Low Testosterone

About one-half of XXY males' chromosomes have low testosterone levels. These levels can be raised by taking supplemental testosterone. Testosterone treatment can:

- Improve muscle mass
- Deepen the voice
- Promote growth of facial and body hair
- Help the reproductive organs to mature
- Build and maintain bone strength and help prevent osteoporosis in later years
- Produce a more masculine appearance, which can also help relieve anxiety and depression
- Increase focus and attention

There are various ways to take testosterone:

- injections or shots, every 2 to 3 weeks
- pills
- through the skin, also called transdermal; current methods include wearing a testosterone patch or rubbing testosterone gel on the skin

Males taking testosterone treatment should work closely with an endocrinologist, a doctor who specializes in hormones and their functions, to ensure the best outcome from testosterone therapy.

Is Testosterone Therapy Right For Every XXY Male?

Not all males with XXY condition benefit from testosterone therapy.

For males whose testosterone level is low to normal, the benefits of taking testosterone are less clear than for when testosterone is very low. Side effects, although generally mild, can include acne, skin rashes from patches or gels, breathing problems (especially during sleep), and higher risk of an enlarged prostate gland or prostate cancer in older age. In addition, testosterone supplementation will not increase testicular size, decrease breast growth, or correct infertility.

Although the majority of boys with KS grow up to live as males, some develop atypical gender identities. For these males, supplemental testosterone may not be suitable. Gender identity should be discussed with healthcare specialists before starting treatment.

Treating Language And Learning Symptoms

Some, but not all, children with KS have language development and learning delays. They might be slow to learn to talk, read, and write, and they might have difficulty processing what they hear. But various interventions, such as speech therapy and educational assistance, can help to reduce and even eliminate these difficulties. The earlier treatment begins, the better the outcomes.

Parents might need to bring these types of problems to the teacher's attention. Because these boys can be quiet and cooperative in the classroom, teachers may not notice the need for help.

Boys and men with KS can benefit by visiting therapists who are experts in areas such as coordination, social skills, and coping. XXY males might benefit from any or all of the following:

- physical therapists
- occupational therapists
- behavioral therapists
- mental health therapists or counselors
- family therapists

Parents of XXY males have also mentioned that taking part in physical activities at low-key levels, such as karate, swimming, tennis, and golf, were helpful in improving motor skills, coordination, and confidence.

With regard to education, some boys with KS will qualify to receive state-sponsored special needs services to address their developmental and learning symptoms. But, because these symptoms may be mild, many XXY males will not be eligible for these services.

Treating Social And Behavioral Symptoms

Many of the professionals and methods for treating learning and language symptoms of the XXY condition are similar to or the same as the ones used to address social and behavioral symptoms.

For instance, boys with KS may need help with social skills and interacting in groups. Occupational or behavioral therapists might be able to assist with these skills. Some school districts and health centers might also offer these types of skill-building programs or classes.

In adolescence, symptoms such as lack of body hair could make XXY males uncomfortable in school or other social settings, and this discomfort can lead to depression, substance abuse, and behavioral problems or "acting out." They might also have questions about their masculinity or gender identity. In these instances, consulting a psychologist, counselor, or psychiatrist may be helpful.

How Do Healthcare Providers Diagnose Klinefelter Syndrome

The only way to confirm the presence of an extra chromosome is by a karyotype test. A healthcare provider will take a small blood or skin sample and send it to a laboratory, where a technician inspects the cells under a microscope to find the extra chromosome. A karyotype test shows the same results at any time in a person's life.

Tests for chromosome disorders, including KS, may be done before birth. To obtain tissue or liquid for this test, a pregnant woman undergoes chorionic villus sampling or amniocentesis. These types of prenatal testing carry a small risk for miscarriage and are not routinely conducted unless the woman has a family history of chromosomal disorders, has other medical problems, or is above 35 years of age.

Factors That Influence When Klinefelter Syndrome Is Diagnosed

Because symptoms can be mild, some males with KS are never diagnosed.

Several factors affect whether and when a diagnosis occurs:

- Few newborns and boys are tested for or diagnosed with KS.

  - Although newborns in the United States are screened for some conditions, they are not screened for XXY or other sex-chromosome differences.

  - In childhood, symptoms can be subtle and overlooked easily. Only about 1 in 10 males with KS is diagnosed before puberty.

  - Sometimes, visiting a healthcare provider will not produce a diagnosis. Some symptoms, such as delayed early speech, might be treated successfully without further testing for KS.

- Most XXY diagnoses occur at puberty or in adulthood.

  - Puberty brings a surge in diagnoses as some males (or their parents) become concerned about slow testes growth or breast development and consult a healthcare provider.

  - Many men are diagnosed for the first time in fertility clinics. Among men seeking help for infertility, about 15 percent have KS

Is There A Cure For Klinefelter Syndrome

Currently, there is no way to remove chromosomes from cells to "cure" the XXY condition.

But many symptoms can be successfully treated, minimizing the impact the condition has on length and quality of life. Most adult XXY men have full independence and have friends, families, and normal social relationships. They live about as long as other men, on average.

Chapter 32

Turner Syndrome

Turner syndrome is a chromosomal disorder that affects development in females. It results when a female's cells has one normal X chromosome and the other X chromosome is either missing or structurally altered (females without Turner syndrome have two normal X chromosomes in each cell). Signs and symptoms may include short stature; premature ovarian failure; a "webbed" neck; a low hairline at the back of the neck; and swelling (lymphedema) of the hands and feet. Some people with Turner syndrome have skeletal abnormalities, kidney problems, and/or a congenital heart defect. Treatment may include growth hormone therapy for short stature and estrogen therapy to help stimulate sexual development.

Symptoms

There are various signs and symptoms of Turner syndrome, which can range from very mild to more severe. Short stature is the most common feature and usually becomes apparent by age 5. In early childhood, frequent middle ear infections are common and can lead to hearing loss in some cases. Most affected girls do not produce the necessary sex hormones for puberty, so they don't have a pubertal growth spurt, start their periods or develop breasts without hormone treatment. While most affected women are infertile, pregnancy is possible with egg donation and assisted reproductive technology. Intelligence is usually normal, but developmental delay, learning disabilities, and/or behavioral problems are sometimes present.

About This Chapter: This chapter includes text excerpted from "Turner Syndrome," Genetic and Rare Diseases Information Center (GARD), National Center for Advancing Translational Sciences (NCATS), 2016.

Additional symptoms of Turner syndrome may include:

- a wide, webbed neck

- a low or indistinct hairline in the back of the head

- swelling (lymphedema) of the hands and feet

- broad chest and widely spaced nipples

- arms that turn out slightly at the elbow

- congenital heart defects or heart murmur

- scoliosis (curving of the spine) or other skeletal abnormalities

- kidney problems

- an underactive thyroid gland

- a slightly increased risk to develop diabetes, especially if older or overweight

- osteoporosis due to a lack of estrogen (usually prevented by hormone replacement therapy)

Cause

Turner syndrome is caused by partial or complete loss of one of the X chromosomes in cells of females. Females without Turner syndrome have 2 full X chromosome in all of their cells (and males have one X chromosome and one Y chromosome). The missing genetic material affects development before and after birth.

Most females with Turner syndrome are missing a full X chromosome in all of their cells (also called monosomy X). This form results from a random error in an egg or sperm cell prior to conception.

Some females with Turner syndrome have two X chromosomes, but one of them is missing a piece (has a deletion). Depending on the specific gene(s) that are missing, the features of Turner syndrome may result. A deletion may occur sporadically (not inherited) or may be inherited from a parent.

Mosaic Turner syndrome (when some cells have one X chromosome and some have two sex chromosomes) is caused by a random error in early fetal development (shortly after conception).

It is still unclear exactly which genes on the X chromosome are associated with each feature of Turner syndrome. It is known that the *SHOX* gene on the X chromosome is important for growth and bone development. A missing copy of this gene is thought to result in the short stature and skeletal abnormalities in many affected women.

Inheritance

Most cases of Turner syndrome are not inherited. Most commonly, Turner syndrome occurs due to a random event during the formation of an egg or sperm cell in a parent (prior to conception). For example, if an egg or sperm cell mistakenly loses a sex chromosome, and joins at conception with an egg or sperm containing an X chromosome, the resulting child will have a single X chromosome in each cell.

Mosaic Turner syndrome, occurring when a person has some cells with one X chromosome and some cells with two X chromosomes, is also not inherited. This also occurs due to a random event, during early fetal development rather than before conception.

In rare cases, Turner syndrome may be caused by a missing piece (partial deletion) of the X chromosome. A deletion can be inherited from a parent.

Genetic testing of an affected fetus or child can identify the type of Turner syndrome present and may help to estimate the risk of recurrence. People with questions about genetic testing or recurrence risks for Turner syndrome are encouraged to speak with a genetics professional.

Treatment

FDA-Approved Treatments

The medication(s) listed below have been approved by the U.S. Food and Drug Administration (FDA) as orphan products for treatment of this condition.

- **Somatropin (Brand name: Humatrope)**

   FDA-approved indication: Treatment of short stature associated with Turner syndrome in patients whose epiphyses are not closed.

- **Somatropin (r-DNA) for injection (Brand name: Nutropin®)**

   FDA-approved indication: Treatment of children with growth failure associated with chronic renal insufficiency.

Prognosis

The long-term outlook (prognosis) for people with Turner syndrome is typically good. Life expectancy is slightly shorter than average but may be improved by addressing and treating associated chronic illnesses, such as obesity and hypertension. Regular checkups have shown substantial improvements in the quality and length of life for women with Turner syndrome. While almost all women are infertile, pregnancy with donor eggs and assisted reproductive technology is possible. Even with growth hormone therapy, most affected people are shorter than average.

Other Names

- Ullrich-Turner syndrome

- Bonnevie-Ulrich syndrome

- 45,X Syndrome

- Chromosome X Monosomy X

- Gonadal Dysgenesis (45,X)

- Schereshevkii Turner Syndrome

- Turner Varny Syndrome

Part Five
Academic Issues

Chapter 33
Choosing A School

Today there is a dizzying array of options available when it comes to choosing a school for students with learning disabilities (LD). These range from regular classrooms with trained staff support to ordinary schools with dedicated special-needs programs to specialized schools for LD students. Although this is certainly a good thing, it also creates a daunting task for parents and teens attempting to sort through the choices.

The first step is to have the student's LD properly assessed, if this has not already been done. An accurate evaluation is necessary in order to focus on those schools or programs that are best suited to the student's particular needs. Testing can be done through public programs or privately by a licensed professional—usually a clinical psychologist, an educational psychologist, or a neuropsychologist—and generally consists of evaluating overall intelligence, memory, reasoning, achievement and ability in various areas, verbal skills, and physical ability.

Before the passage of The Individuals with Disabilities Education Act (IDEA) (formerly called the Education for All Handicapped Children Act), just one in five students with physical, psychological, or learning disabilities were being educated in U.S. schools. This legislation requires that all students receive free access to an appropriate education.

(Source: " A 25 Year History Of The IDEA," U.S. Department of Education (ED).)

"Choosing A School," © 2017 Omnigraphics. Reviewed December 2016.

Types Of Schools For LD Students

Once the assessment process is complete, the professionals who analyzed the results will go over their findings and can help with recommendations for the type of school that is most appropriate for the student. These may include:

- **Public schools.** Neighborhood schools have several immediate advantages: they're close to home, are free, and allow the teen to interact with many different types of students. They are also required by law to give the student an appropriate education, which means helping develop an appropriate program to meet his or her needs. This can include special support in a regular classroom, dedicated classes for students with similar needs, and specially trained staff. But public schools can vary considerably in available resources for LD students, and possible downsides include less individual attention due to large class sizes and few special-education teachers on staff.

- **Charter schools and magnet schools.** These still operate under the public-school system, which means there is no charge to attend. Some focus on specific areas of education, so it's possible to select one that aligns with the student's academic strengths, yet they also provide support for those with learning disabilities. In addition, the class sizes tend to be smaller, and some of these schools even focus specifically on LD students. On the other hand, they may not be near the student's home, can have waiting lists for admission, and, in the case of charter schools, which are run by private or community groups, might have limited funding available for LD education.

- **Private schools.** Private schools almost always have smaller class sizes, which allows for more individual attention. They can also provide a different type of education than is found in public schools, such as religious instruction or a focus on specific subjects. And although private schools are not required by law to provide services to LD students, some may be equipped to do so, and in other cases, the student might be eligible to receive these services through the local public school. Of course, private schools charge tuition, which may be very expensive, although scholarships and financial aid could be available.

- **Private schools for LD students.** Most LD students attend ordinary schools, but some want or need a school that specializes in teaching students with their disability. These schools are able to provide the most support, with teachers and staff who have the most comprehensive training, as well as curricula and programs that have been specifically designed for LD students. In addition, the environment is generally more welcoming to individuals with disabilities, and other students tend to be more accepting of their peers.

However, in this type of school, the student's interaction will be limited to others with learning disabilities, which can be a drawback to social development. And, again, tuition can be expensive, but in some cases, the local school system might assume the expense if it is not able to provide an appropriate education elsewhere.

- **Homeschooling.** Although it's not for everyone, homeschooling can provide certain advantages for both parents and students. For example, individual attention is maximized, coursework can be tailored to the student's needs, and some issues, like bullying, can be eliminated. Of course homeschooling requires an intense commitment—in both time and energy—on the part of the parent or other person who will be responsible for the LD student's education. There's also the need to ensure that the student interacts regularly with other individuals his or her own age through outside activities.

Steps In Choosing A School

Once the type of school has been determined, based on the particular needs and preferences of the LD student and parents, the next task is to decide on a specific school. Some steps include:

- **Gather information.** The phone book might be one place to start. But a more focused plan might be to ask for recommendations from the health or educational professional who currently works with the LD student, from another parent or student, or from the local chapter of the Learning Disabilities Association of America.

- **Narrow down the choices.** This is a good time to use the Internet or consult published sources for pluses and minuses about the various schools under consideration. It's also a good idea to collect pamphlets or other written information from various schools, check school ratings and evaluations, and even attend parent fairs and open houses. If possible, talk to parents and students who are familiar with these schools for personal opinions.

- **Investigate the school.** Once a potential choice has been identified, it's time to burrow down into the details. Find out if the school is properly accredited, read the school's mission statement (usually available on its web site), explore teacher requirements and certifications, learn about special programs and extracurricular activities that might benefit the student. And, finally, visit the school, ideally more than once. Observe a typical day, get a feel for the environment, check out the classrooms and see what technology is in use there, and, if possible, sit in on a class or two. Meet with the head of the school, some of the teachers, and, if this can be arranged, a current student and his or her parents. Ask as many questions as possible about the curriculum, teaching methods, programs and facilities devoted to the student's particular LD, the school's daily routine, how behavioral issues are handled, communication style, family involvement, and any other areas of concern.

> The field of special education is constantly evolving, so schools need to ensure that teachers are up to date on the latest research and methods. Before deciding on a school, ask about its program for the ongoing development of staff.

References

1 Blake, Hannah. "Choosing the Right School for Your Child With Learning Difficulties or a Learning Disability," MadeForMums.com, n.d.

2 Chaban, Peter. "Choosing the Right School for Special Needs Children," AboutKidsHealth.ca, September 3, 2010.

3 Dwight, Valle. "Special Needs Programs and Schools: A Primer," GreatSchools.org, April 30, 2015.

4 Tucker, Geri Coleman. "Choosing a School: Know the Options for Your Child," Understood.org, Mar 30, 2014.

5 Weston, Susan Perkins, with Joe Nathan and Mary Anne Raywid. "Choosing a School for Your Child," Office of Educational Research and Improvement, U.S. Department of Education, 2005.

Chapter 34

Evaluating And Documenting A Learning Disability

The Purpose Of Evaluation: Finding Out Why

Many children have trouble in school. Some have trouble learning to read or write. Others have a hard time remembering new information. Still others may have trouble behaving themselves. Children can have all sorts of problems.

It's important to find out why a child is not doing well in school. The child may have a disability. By law, schools must provide special help to eligible children with disabilities. This help is called special education and related services.

You may ask the school to evaluate your child, or the school may ask you for permission to do an evaluation. If the school thinks your child may have a disability and may need special education and related services, the school must evaluate your child before providing your child with these services. This evaluation is at no cost to you.

Once you give your informed written permission for the evaluation, the school has 60 days to evaluate your child. (If your state has set its own timeframe for conducting evaluations, then the school will follow the state's timeframe.) The evaluation will tell you and the school:

- if your child has a disability; and

- what kind of special help your child needs in school.

About This Chapter: Text under the heading "The Purpose Of Evaluation: Finding Out Why" is excerpted from "Your Child's Evaluation," Center for Parent Information and Resources (CPIR), U.S. Department of Education (ED), 2009. Reviewed December 2016; Text under the heading "Documentation Required For The Eligibility Determination" is excerpted from "Identification Of Specific Learning Disabilities," U.S. Department of Education (ED), September 1, 2006. Reviewed December 2016.

Step 1: Using What Is Known

A team of people, including you, will be involved in evaluating your child. This team will begin by looking at what is already known about your child. The team will look at your child's school file and recent test scores. You and your child's teacher(s) may provide information to be included in this review.

The evaluation team needs enough information to decide if your child has a disability. It also needs to know what kind of special help your child needs. Is there enough information about your child to answer these questions? If your child is being evaluated for the first time, maybe not.

Step 2: Collecting More Information

The team of people involved in your child's evaluation, including you, will identify what additional information about your child is needed in order to answer the questions we just mentioned. Before the school may conduct additional testing to collect that information, school personnel must ask you for permission. They must explain to you what the evaluation of your child will involve. This includes describing (a) the tests they will use with your child, and (b) the other ways they will collect information about your child.

The school will collect the additional information about your child in many different ways and from many different people, including you. Tests are an important part of an evaluation, but they are only one part. The evaluation should also include:

- the observations and opinions of professionals who have worked with your child;

- your child's medical history, when it's relevant to his or her performance in school; and

- your observations about your child's experiences, abilities, needs, and behavior in school and outside of school, and his or her feelings about school.

Who Is Involved In Your Child's Evaluation?

The team involved in your child's evaluation will include these people:

- you, as parents or guardians;
- at least one of your child's regular education teachers (if your child is, or may be, participating in the regular education environment);
- at least one of your child's special education teachers or service providers;

- a school administrator who knows about policies for special education, children with disabilities, available resources, and the general curriculum (the curriculum used by children without disabilities);
- someone who can explain the evaluation results and talk about what instruction may be necessary for your child;
- your child, if appropriate;
- representatives from other agencies that may be responsible for paying for or providing transition services (if your child is 16 years, or younger, if appropriate);
- individuals (invited by you or the school) with knowledge or special expertise about your child, including related service providers (such as a speech therapist, physical therapist, or school nurse); and
- other qualified professionals, as appropriate (such as a behavioral or medical specialist).

Professionals will observe your child. They may give your child tests. They are trying to get a picture of the "whole child." It's important that the school evaluate your child in all areas where he or she might have a disability. For example, they will want to know more about:

- how well your child speaks and understands language;
- how your child thinks and behaves;
- how well your child adapts to change;
- what your child has achieved in school;
- how well your child functions in areas such as movement, thinking, learning, seeing, and hearing; and
- what job-related and other postschool interests and abilities your child has (important when your child is nearing 16 years old, or sooner, if appropriate).

Evaluating your child completely will help you and the school decide if your child has a disability. The information will also help you and the school plan instruction for your child.

Step 3: Deciding If Your Child Is Eligible For Special Education

The next step is to decide if your child is eligible for special education and related services. This decision will be based on the results of your child's evaluation and the policies in your area about eligibility for these special services.

It's important that your child's evaluation results be explained to you in a way that's easy to understand. The school will discuss your child's scores on tests and what they mean. Is your child doing as well as other children his or her age? What does your child do well? Where is your child having trouble? What is causing the trouble?

If you don't understand something in your child's evaluation results, be sure to speak up and ask questions. This is your child. You know your child very well. Do the results make sense, considering what you know about your child? Share your special insights. Your knowledge of your child is important.

Based on your child's evaluation results, a group of people will decide if your child is eligible for special education and related services. Under Individuals with Disabilities Education Act (IDEA), you have the right to be part of any group that decides your child's eligibility for special education and related services.

This decision is based in part on IDEA's definition of a "child with a disability." You should know that:

- The IDEA lists 13 different disability categories under which a child may be eligible for services.

- The disability must affect the child's educational performance. (Your child does not have to be failing school, however, and may be moving from grade to grade.)

- A child may not be identified as having a disability primarily because he or she speaks a language other than English and does not speak or understand English well. A child may not be identified as having a disability just because he or she has not had enough appropriate instruction in math or reading.

As a parent, you have the right to receive a copy of the evaluation report on your child at no cost to you. You also have the right to receive a copy of the paperwork about your child's eligibility for special education and related services.

Individuals with Disabilities Education Act (IDEA)

Our country's special education law is called the Individuals with Disabilities Education Act (IDEA). The IDEA is a very important law for children with disabilities, their families, and schools. The evaluation process described here is based on what this law requires.

IDEA's Categories Of Disability

- Autism

- Deaf-blindness
- Deafness
- Hearing impairment
- Intellectual disability
- Multiple disabilities
- Orthopedic impairment
- Other health impairment (i.e., having limited strength, vitality, or alertness that affects a child's educational performance)
- Serious emotional disturbance
- Specific learning disability
- Speech or language impairment
- Traumatic brain injury
- Visual impairment, including blindness

If your child is eligible for special education and related services (such as speech therapy) and you agree with this determination, then you and the school will meet and talk about your child's special educational needs. However, you can disagree with the decision and refuse special education and related services for your child.

If your child is not eligible for special education and related services, the school must tell you so in writing. You must also receive information about what to do if you disagree with this decision. If this information is not in the materials the school gives you, ask for it. You have the right to disagree with the eligibility decision and be heard. Also, ask how the school will help your child if he or she will not be getting special education services.

Four Evaluation "Musts"

- **Using the native language:** The evaluation must be conducted in your child's native language (for example, Spanish) or other means of communication (for example, sign language, if your child is deaf), unless it clearly isn't possible to do so.
- **No discrimination:** Each test must be given in a way that does not discriminate against your child because he or she has a disability or is from a different racial or cultural background.
- **Trained evaluators:** The people who test your child must know how to give the tests they decide to use. They must give each test according to the instructions that came with the test.

> • **More than one procedure:** Evaluation results will be used to decide if your child is a "child with a disability" and to determine what kind of educational program your child needs. These decisions cannot be made based on only one procedure such as only one test.

Step 4: Developing Your Child's Educational Program

If, however, your child is found eligible for special education and related services and you agree, the next step is to write an Individualized Education Program (IEP) for your child. This is a written document that you and school personnel develop together. The IEP will describe your child's educational program, including the special services your child will receive.

Documentation Required For The Eligibility Determination

For a child suspected of having a specific learning disability, the documentation of the determination of eligibility, as required in 34 CFR 300.306(a)(2), must contain a statement of:

- Whether the child has a specific learning disability;

- The basis for making the determination, including an assurance that the determination has been made in accordance with 34 CFR 300.306(c)(1);

- The relevant behavior, if any, noted during the observation of the child and the relationship of that behavior to the child's academic functioning;

- The educationally relevant medical findings, if any;

- Whether the child does not achieve adequately for the child's age or to meet State-approved grade-level standards consistent with 34 CFR 300.309(a)(1); and the child does not make sufficient progress to meet age or State-approved grade-level standards consistent with 34 CFR 300.309(a)(2)(i); or the child exhibits a pattern of strengths and weaknesses in performance, achievement, or both, relative to age, State-approved grade level standards or intellectual development consistent with 34 CFR 300.309(a)(2)(i); or the child exhibits a pattern of strengths and weaknesses in performance, achievement, or both, relative to age, State-approved grade-level standards or intellectual development consistent with 34 CFR 300.309(a)(2)(ii);

- The determination of the group concerning the effects of a visual, hearing, or motor disability; mental retardation; emotional disturbance; cultural factors; environmental or economic disadvantage; or limited English proficiency on the child's achievement level; and

- If the child has participated in a process that assesses the child's response to scientific, research-based intervention:

- The instructional strategies used and the student-centered data collected; and

- The documentation that the child's parents were notified about: (1) the State's policies regarding the amount and nature of student performance data that would be collected and the general education services that would be provided; (2) strategies for increasing the child's rate of learning; and (3) the parents' right to request an evaluation.

Each group member must certify in writing whether the report reflects the member's conclusion. If it does not reflect the member's conclusion, the group member must submit a separate statement presenting the member's conclusions.

Chapter 35

The Individualized Education Plan (IEP)

What's An Individualized Education Program (IEP)?

Kids with delayed skills or other disabilities might be eligible for special services that provide individualized education programs in public schools, free of charge to families. Understanding how to access these services can help parents be effective advocates for their kids.

The passage of the updated version of the Individuals with Disabilities Education Act (IDEA 2004) made parents of kids with special needs even more crucial members of their child's education team.

Parents can now work with educators to develop a plan—the individualized education program (IEP)—to help kids succeed in school. The IEP describes the goals the team sets for a child during the school year, as well as any special support needed to help achieve them.

Who Needs An IEP?

A child who has difficulty learning and functioning and has been identified as a special needs student is the perfect candidate for an IEP.

Kids struggling in school may qualify for support services, allowing them to be taught in a special way, for reasons such as:

- learning disabilities

- attention deficit hyperactivity disorder (ADHD)

- emotional disorders

- cognitive challenges

- autism

- hearing impairment

- visual impairment

- speech or language impairment

- developmental delay

- physical disabilities

How Are Services Delivered?

In most cases, the services and goals outlined in an IEP can be provided in a standard school environment. This can be done in the regular classroom (for example, a reading teacher helping a small group of children who need extra assistance while the other kids in the class work on reading with the regular teacher) or in a special resource room in the regular school. The resource room can serve a group of kids with similar needs who are brought together for help.

However, kids who need intense intervention may be taught in a special school environment. These classes have fewer students per teacher, allowing for more individualized attention.

In addition, the teacher usually has specific training in helping kids with special educational needs. The children spend most of their day in a special classroom and join the regular classes for nonacademic activities (like music and gym) or in academic activities in which they don't need extra help.

Because the goal of IDEA is to ensure that each child is educated in the least restrictive environment possible, effort is made to help kids stay in a regular classroom. However, when needs are best met in a special class, then kids might be placed in one.

The Referral And Evaluation Process

The referral process generally begins when a teacher, parent, or doctor is concerned that a child may be having trouble in the classroom, and the teacher notifies the school counselor or psychologist.

The first step is to gather specific data regarding the student's progress or academic problems. This may be done through:

- a conference with parents

- a conference with the student

- observation of the student
- analysis of the student's performance (attention, behavior, work completion, tests, classwork, homework, etc.)

This information helps school personnel determine the next step. At this point, strategies specific to the student could be used to help the child become more successful in school. If this doesn't work, the child would be tested for a specific learning disability or other impairment to help determine qualification for special services.

It's important to note, though, that the presence of a disability doesn't automatically guarantee a child will receive services. To be eligible, the disability must affect functioning at school.

To determine eligibility, a multidisciplinary team of professionals will evaluate the child based on their observations; the child's performance on standardized tests; and daily work such as tests, quizzes, classwork, and homework.

Who's On The Team?

The professionals on the evaluation team can include:

- a psychologist
- a physical therapist
- an occupational therapist
- a speech therapist
- a special educator
- a vision or hearing specialist
- others, depending on the child's specific needs

As a parent, you can decide whether to have your child assessed. If you choose to do so, you'll be asked to sign a permission form that will detail who is involved in the process and the types of tests they use. These tests might include measures of specific school skills, such as reading or math, as well as more general developmental skills, such as speech and language. Testing does not necessarily mean that a child will receive services.

Once the team members complete their individual assessments, they develop a comprehensive evaluation report (CER) that compiles their findings, offers an educational classification, and outlines the skills and support the child will need.

The parents then have a chance to review the report before the IEP is developed. Some parents will disagree with the report, and they will have the opportunity to work together with the school to come up with a plan that best meets the child's needs.

Developing An IEP

The next step is an IEP meeting at which the team and parents decide what will go into the plan. In addition to the evaluation team, a regular teacher should be present to offer suggestions about how the plan can help the child's progress in the standard education curriculum.

At the meeting, the team will discuss your child's educational needs—as described in the CER—and come up with specific, measurable short-term and annual goals for each of those needs. If you attend this meeting, you can take an active role in developing the goals and determining which skills or areas will receive the most attention.

The cover page of the IEP outlines the support services your child will receive and how often they will be provided (for example, occupational therapy twice a week). Support services might include special education, speech therapy, occupational or physical therapy, counseling, audiology, medical services, nursing, and vision or hearing therapy. They might also include transportation; the extent of participation in programs for students without disabilities; what, if any, modifications are needed in the administration of statewide assessment of student achievement; and, beginning at age 14, the inclusion of transition planning as a part of the process.

If the team recommends several services, the amount of time they take in the child's school schedule can seem overwhelming. To ease that load, some services may be provided on a consultative basis. In these cases, the professional consults with the teacher to come up with strategies to help the child but doesn't offer any hands-on instruction. For instance, an occupational therapist may suggest accommodations for a child with fine-motor problems that affect handwriting, and the classroom teacher would incorporate these suggestions into the handwriting lessons taught to the entire class.

Other services can be delivered right in the classroom, so the child's day isn't interrupted by therapy. The child who has difficulty with handwriting might work one on one with an occupational therapist while everyone else practices their handwriting skills. When deciding how and where services are offered, the child's comfort and dignity should be a top priority.

The IEP should be reviewed annually to update the goals and make sure the levels of service meet your child's needs. However, IEPs can be changed at any time on an as-needed basis.

If you think your child needs more, fewer, or different services, you can request a meeting and bring the team together to discuss your concerns.

Your Legal Rights

Specific timelines ensure that the development of an IEP moves from referral to providing services as quickly as possible. Be sure to ask about this timeframe and get a copy of your parents' rights when your child is referred. These guidelines (sometimes called procedural safeguards) outline your rights as a parent to control what happens to your child during each step of the process.

The parents' rights also describe how you can proceed if you disagree with any part of the CER or the IEP—mediation and hearings both are options. You can get information about low-cost or free legal representation from the school district or, if your child is in Early Intervention (for kids up to age 3), through that program.

Attorneys and paid advocates familiar with the IEP process will provide representation if you need it. You also may invite anyone who knows or works with your child whose input you feel would be helpful to join the IEP team. Federally supported programs in each state support parent-to-parent information and training activities for parents of children with special needs. The Parent Training and Information Projects conduct workshops, publish newsletters, and answer questions by phone or by mail about parent-to-parent activities.

A Final Word

Parents have the right to choose where their kids will be educated. This choice includes public or private elementary schools and secondary schools, including religious schools. It also includes charter schools and home schools.

However, it is important to understand that the rights of children with disabilities who are placed by their parents in private elementary schools and secondary schools are not the same as those of kids with disabilities who are enrolled in public schools or placed by public agencies in private schools when the public school is unable to provide a free appropriate public education (FAPE).

Two major differences that parents, teachers, other school staff, private school representatives, and the kids need to know about are:

- Children with disabilities who are placed by their parents in private schools may not get the same services they would receive in a public school.

- Not all kids with disabilities placed by their parents in private schools will receive services.

The IEP process is complex, but it's also an effective way to address how your child learns and functions. If you have concerns, don't hesitate to ask questions about the evaluation findings or the goals recommended by the team. You know your child best and should play a central role in creating a learning plan tailored to his or her specific needs.

Chapter 36

Effective Academic Instruction For Children With ADHD

Academic Instruction

The first major component of the most effective instruction for children with attention deficit hyperactivity disorder (ADHD) is effective academic instruction. Teachers can help prepare their students with ADHD to achieve by applying the principles of effective teaching when they introduce, conduct, and conclude each lesson.

Introducing Lessons

Students with ADHD learn best with a carefully structured academic lesson-one where the teacher explains what he or she wants children to learn in the current lesson and places these skills and knowledge in the context of previous lessons. Effective teachers preview their expectations about what students will learn and how they should behave during the lesson. A number of teaching-related practices have been found especially useful in facilitating this process:

- **Provide an advance organizer.**

  Prepare students for the day's lesson by quickly summarizing the order of various activities planned. Explain, for example, that a review of the previous lesson will be followed by new information and that both group and independent work will be expected.

About This Chapter: This chapter includes text excerpted from "Teaching Children With Attention Deficit Hyperactivity Disorder: Instructional Strategies And Practices," U.S. Department of Education (ED), October 3, 2008. Reviewed December 2016.

- **Review previous lessons.**

  Review information about previous lessons on this topic. For example, remind children that yesterday's lesson focused on learning how to regroup in subtraction. Review several problems before describing the current lesson.

- **Set learning expectations.**

  State what students are expected to learn during the lesson. For example, explain to students that a language arts lesson will involve reading a story about Paul Bunyan and identifying new vocabulary words in the story.

- **Set behavioral expectations.**

  Describe how students are expected to behave during the lesson. For example, tell children that they may talk quietly to their neighbors as they do their seatwork or they may raise their hands to get your attention.

- **State needed materials.**

  Identify all materials that the children will need during the lesson, rather than leaving them to figure out on their own the materials required. For example, specify that children need their journals and pencils for journal writing or their crayons, scissors, and colored paper for an art project.

- **Explain additional resources.**

  Tell students how to obtain help in mastering the lesson. For example, refer children to a particular page in the textbook for guidance on completing a worksheet.

- **Simplify instructions, choices, and scheduling.**

  The simpler the expectations communicated to an ADHD student, the more likely it is that he or she will comprehend and complete them in a timely and productive manner.

Conducting Lessons

In order to conduct the most productive lessons for children with ADHD, effective teachers periodically question children's understanding of the material, probe for correct answers before calling on other students, and identify which students need additional assistance. Teachers should keep in mind that transitions from one lesson or class to another are particularly difficult for students with ADHD. When they are prepared for transitions, these children are more likely to respond and to stay on task. The following set of strategies may assist teachers in conducting effective lessons:

- **Be predictable.**

  Structure and consistency are very important for children with ADHD; many do not deal well with change. Minimal rules and minimal choices are best for these children. They need to understand clearly what is expected of them, as well as the consequences for not adhering to expectations.

- **Support the student's participation in the classroom.**

  Provide students with ADHD with private, discreet cues to stay on task and advance warning that they will be called upon shortly. Avoid bringing attention to differences between ADHD students and their classmates. At all times, avoid the use of sarcasm and criticism.

- **Use audiovisual materials.**

  Use a variety of audiovisual materials to present academic lessons. For example, use an overhead projector to demonstrate how to solve an addition problem requiring regrouping. The students can work on the problem at their desks while you manipulate counters on the projector screen.

- **Check student performance.**

  Question individual students to assess their mastery of the lesson. For example, you can ask students doing seatwork (i.e., lessons completed by students at their desks in the classroom) to demonstrate how they arrived at the answer to a problem, or you can ask individual students to state, in their own words, how the main character felt at the end of the story.

- **Ask probing questions.**

  Probe for the correct answer after allowing a child sufficient time to work out the answer to a question. Count at least 15 seconds before giving the answer or calling on another student. Ask follow-up questions that give children an opportunity to demonstrate what they know.

- **Perform ongoing student evaluation.**

  Identify students who need additional assistance. Watch for signs of lack of comprehension, such as daydreaming or visual or verbal indications of frustration. Provide these children with extra explanations, or ask another student to serve as a peer tutor for the lesson.

- **Help students correct their own mistakes.**

  Describe how students can identify and correct their own mistakes. For example, remind students that they should check their calculations in math problems and reiterate how they can check their calculations; remind students of particularly difficult spelling rules and how students can watch out for easy-to-make errors.

- **Help students focus.**

  Remind students to keep working and to focus on their assigned task. For example, you can provide follow-up directions or assign learning partners. These practices can be directed at individual children or at the entire class.

- **Follow-up directions.**

  Effective teachers of children with ADHD also guide them with follow-up directions:

  - *Oral directions:* After giving directions to the class as a whole, provide additional oral directions for a child with ADHD. For example, ask the child if he or she understood the directions and repeat the directions together.

  - *Written directions.* Provide follow-up directions in writing. For example, write the page number for an assignment on the chalkboard and remind the child to look at the chalkboard if he or she forgets the assignment.

- **Lower noise level.**

  Monitor the noise level in the classroom, and provide corrective feedback, as needed. If the noise level exceeds the level appropriate for the type of lesson, remind all students or individual students about the behavioral rules stated at the beginning of the lesson.

- **Divide work into smaller units.**

  Break down assignments into smaller, less complex tasks. For example, allow students to complete five math problems before presenting them with the remaining five problems.

- **Highlight key points.**

  Highlight key words in the instructions on worksheets to help the child with ADHD focus on the directions. Prepare the worksheet before the lesson begins, or underline key words as you and the child read the directions together. When reading, show children how to identify and highlight a key sentence, or have them write it on a separate piece of paper, before asking for a summary of the entire book. In math, show children how to underline the important facts and operations; in "Mary has two apples, and John has three," underline "two," "and," and "three."

- **Eliminate or reduce frequency of timed tests.**

  Tests that are timed may not allow children with ADHD to demonstrate what they truly know due to their potential preoccupation with elapsed time. Allow students with ADHD more time to complete quizzes and tests in order to eliminate "test anxiety," and provide them with other opportunities, methods, or test formats to demonstrate their knowledge.

- **Use cooperative learning strategies.**

  Have students work together in small groups to maximize their own and each other's learning. Use strategies such as Think-Pair-Share where teachers ask students to think about a topic, pair with a partner to discuss it, and share ideas with the group.

- **Use assistive technology.**

  All students, and those with ADHD in particular, can benefit from the use of technology (such as computers and projector screens), which makes instruction more visual and allows students to participate actively.

Concluding Lessons

Effective teachers conclude their lessons by providing advance warning that the lesson is about to end, checking the completed assignments of at least some of the students with ADHD, and instructing students how to begin preparing for the next activity.

- **Provide advance warnings.**

  Provide advance warning that a lesson is about to end. Announce 5 or 10 minutes before the end of the lesson (particularly for seatwork and group projects) how much time remains. You may also want to tell students at the beginning of the lesson how much time they will have to complete it.

- **Check assignments.**

  Check completed assignments for at least some students. Review what they have learned during the lesson to get a sense of how ready the class was for the lesson and how to plan the next lesson.

- **Preview the next lesson.**

  Instruct students on how to begin preparing for the next lesson. For example, inform children that they need to put away their textbooks and come to the front of the room for a large-group spelling lesson.

Chapter 37

Individualizing Instructional Practices For Children With ADHD

Effective teachers of students with ADHD individualize their instructional practices in accordance with different academic subjects and the needs of their students within each area. This is because children with ADHD have different ways of learning and retaining information, not all of which involve traditional reading and listening. Effective teachers first identify areas in which each child requires extra assistance and then use special strategies to provide structured opportunities for the child to review and master an academic lesson that was previously presented to the entire class. Strategies that may help facilitate this goal include the following (grouped by subject area):

Language Arts And Reading Comprehension

To help children with attention deficit hyperactivity disorder (ADHD) who are poor readers improve their reading comprehension skills, try the following instructional practices:

- **Silent reading time.**

  Establish a fixed time each day for silent reading (e.g., D.E.A.R.: Drop Everything and Read and Sustained Silent Reading).

- **Follow-along reading.**

  Ask the child to read a story silently while listening to other students or the teacher read the story aloud to the entire class.

About This Chapter: This chapter includes text excerpted from "Teaching Children With Attention Deficit Hyperactivity Disorder: Instructional Strategies And Practices," U.S. Department of Education (ED), October 3, 2008. Reviewed December 2016.

- **Partner reading activities.**

  Pair the child with ADHD with another student partner who is a strong reader. The partners take turns reading orally and listening to each other.

- **Storyboards.**

  Ask the child to make storyboards that illustrate the sequence of main events in a story.

- **Storytelling.**

  Schedule storytelling sessions where the child can retell a story that he or she has read recently.

- **Playacting.**

  Schedule playacting sessions where the child can role-play different characters in a favorite story.

- **Word bank.**

  Keep a word bank or dictionary of new or "hard-to-read" sight-vocabulary words.

- **Board games for reading comprehension.**

  Play board games that provide practice with target reading-comprehension skills or sight-vocabulary words.

- **Computer games for reading comprehension.**

  Schedule computer time for the child to have drill-and-practice with sight vocabulary words.

- **Recorded books.**

  These materials, available from many libraries, can stimulate interest in traditional reading and can be used to reinforce and complement reading lessons.

- **"Backup" materials for home use.**

  Make available to students a second set of books and materials that they can use at home.

- **Summary materials.**

  Allow and encourage students to use published book summaries, synopses, and digests of major reading assignments to review (not replace) reading assignments.

Phonics

To help children with ADHD master rules of phonics, the following are effective:

- **Mnemonics for phonics.**

  Teach the child mnemonics that provide reminders about hard-to-learn phonics rules (e.g., "when two vowels go walking, the first does the talking").

- **Word families.**

  Teach the child to recognize and read word families that illustrate particular phonetic concepts (e.g., "ph" sounds, "at-bat-cat").

- **Board games for phonics.**

  Have students play board games, such as bingo, that allow them to practice phonetically irregular words.

- **Computer games for phonics.**

  Use a computer to provide opportunities for students to drill and practice with phonics or grammar lessons.

- **Picture-letter charts.**

Use these for children who know sounds but do not know the letters that go with them.

Writing

In composing stories or other writing assignments, children with ADHD benefit from the following practices:

- **Standards for writing assignments.**

  Identify and teach the child classroom standards for acceptable written work, such as format and style.

- **Recognizing parts of a story.**

  Teach the student how to describe the major parts of a story (e.g., plot, main characters, setting, conflict, and resolution). Use a storyboard with parts listed for this purpose.

- **Post office.**

  Establish a post office in the classroom, and provide students with opportunities to write, mail, and receive letters to and from their classmates and teacher.

- **Visualize compositions.**

  Ask the child to close his or her eyes and visualize a paragraph that the teacher reads aloud. Another variation of this technique is to ask a student to describe a recent event while the other students close their eyes and visualize what is being said as a written paragraph.

- **Proofread compositions.**

  Require that the child proofread his or her work before turning in written assignments. Provide the child with a list of items to check when proofreading his or her own work.

- **Tape recorders.**

  Ask the student to dictate writing assignments into a tape recorder, as an alternative to writing them.

- **Dictate writing assignments.**

  Have the teacher or another student write down a story told by a child with ADHD.

Spelling

To help children with ADHD who are poor spellers, the following techniques have been found to be helpful:

- **Everyday examples of hard-to-spell words.**

  Take advantage of everyday events to teach difficult spelling words in context. For example, ask a child eating a cheese sandwich to spell "sandwich."

- **Frequently used words.**

  Assign spelling words that the child routinely uses in his or her speech each day.

- **Dictionary of misspelled words.**

  Ask the child to keep a personal dictionary of frequently misspelled words.

- **Partner spelling activities.**

  Pair the child with another student. Ask the partners to quiz each other on the spelling of new words. Encourage both students to guess the correct spelling.

- **Manipulatives.**

  Use cutout letters or other manipulatives to spell out hard-to-learn words.

- **Color-coded letters.**

  Color code different letters in hard-to-spell words (e.g., "receipt").

- **Movement activities.**

  Combine movement activities with spelling lessons (e.g., jump rope while spelling words out loud).

- **Word banks.**

  Use 3" x 5" index cards of frequently misspelled words sorted alphabetically.

Handwriting

Students with ADHD who have difficulty with manuscript or cursive writing may well benefit from their teacher's use of the following instructional practices:

- **Individual chalkboards.**

  Ask the child to practice copying and erasing the target words on a small, individual chalkboard. Two children can be paired to practice their target words together.

- **Quiet places for handwriting.**

  Provide the child with a special "quiet place" (e.g., a table outside the classroom) to complete his or her handwriting assignments.

- **Spacing words on a page.**

  Teach the child to use his or her finger to measure how much space to leave between each word in a written assignment.

- **Special writing paper.**

  Ask the child to use special paper with vertical lines to learn to space letters and words on a page.

- **Structured programs for handwriting.**

  Teach handwriting skills through a structured program.

Math Computation

Numerous individualized instructional practices can help children with ADHD improve their basic computation skills. The following are just a few:

- **Patterns in math.**

  Teach the student to recognize patterns when adding, subtracting, multiplying, or dividing whole numbers. (e.g., the digits of numbers which are multiples of 9 [18, 27, 36 . . .] add up to 9).

- **Partnering for math activities.**

  Pair a child with ADHD with another student and provide opportunities for the partners to quiz each other about basic computation skills.

- **Mastery of math symbols.**

  If children do not understand the symbols used in math, they will not be able to do the work. For instance, do they understand that the "plus" in 1 + 3 means to add and that the "minus" in 5 - 3 means to take away?

- **Mnemonics for basic computation.**

  Teach the child mnemonics that describe basic steps in computing whole numbers. For example, "Don't Miss Susie's Boat" can be used to help the student recall the basic steps in long division (i.e., divide, multiply, subtract, and bring down).

- **Real-life examples of money skills.**

  Provide the child with real-life opportunities to practice target money skills. For example, ask the child to calculate his or her change when paying for lunch in the school cafeteria, or set up a class store where children can practice calculating change.

- **Color coding arithmetic symbols.**

  Color code basic arithmetic symbols, such as +, -, and =, to provide visual cues for children when they are computing whole numbers.

- **Calculators to check basic computation.**

  Ask the child to use a calculator to check addition, subtraction, multiplication, or division.

- **Board games for basic computation.**

  Ask the child to play board games to practice adding, subtracting, multiplying, and dividing whole numbers.

- **Computer games for basic computation.**

  Schedule computer time for the child to drill and practice basic computations, using appropriate games.

- **"Magic minute" drills.**

  Have students perform a quick (60-second) drill every day to practice basic computation of math facts, and have children track their own performance.

Solving Math Word Problems

To help children with ADHD improve their skill in solving word problems in mathematics, try the following:

- **Reread the problem.**

  Teach the child to read a word problem *two times* before beginning to compute the answer.

- **Clue words.**

  Teach the child clue words that identify which operation to use when solving word problems. For example, words such as "sum," "total," or "all together" may indicate an addition operation.

- **Guiding questions for word problems.**

  Teach students to ask guiding questions in solving word problems. For example: What is the question asked in the problem? What information do you need to figure out the answer? What operation should you use to compute the answer?

- **Real-life examples of word problems.**

  Ask the student to create and solve word problems that provide practice with specific target operations, such as addition, subtraction, multiplication, or division. These problems can be based on recent, real-life events in the child's life.

- **Calculators to check word problems.**

  Ask the student to use a calculator to check computations made in answering assigned word problems.

Use Of Special Materials In Math

Some children with ADHD benefit from using special materials to help them complete their math assignments, including:

211

- **Number lines.**

  Provide number lines for the child to use when computing whole numbers.

- **Manipulatives.**

  Use manipulatives to help students gain basic computation skills, such as counting poker chips when adding single-digit numbers.

- **Graph paper.**

  Ask the child to use graph paper to help organize columns when adding, subtracting, multiplying, or dividing whole numbers.

Chapter 38
Improving Study Skills

Homework and studying can be a source of stress for kids and parents alike. Having good study habits in place can reduce that stress. Here are some ideas for improving kids' homework and study skills.

Create A Homework Station

It doesn't matter whether there's a space in your house set aside for homework or a portable homework station. Having a place to keep everything your kid needs for homework can help prevent organization issues and homework battles.

Help your child stock his station with paper, sharpened pencils and other supplies he'll need daily. When he sits down to work, make sure he has enough light and few distractions. And when he's done, have him do a quick check to see if anything needs to be replaced for tomorrow.

Use Checklists

There's something very rewarding about being able to cross a task off a checklist. You can help your child learn how good that feels as well as teach him how to keep track of homework. All he needs is a small pad of paper on which he can list his assignments for the day. As he completes each one, he can cross it off the list.

About This Chapter: Text in this chapter is excerpted from "7 Tips For Improving Your Child's Homework And Study Skills," © 2014–2016 Understood.org USA LLC. Reprinted with permission.

Create A Homework Schedule

A homework schedule can help your child set a specific time for studying (and schedule in breaks between subjects). Help your kid find a time of day when he's able to concentrate, when you're available to help and when he's not in a hurry to get somewhere else.

A homework schedule can also help him keep track of long-term assignments and upcoming tests. Use a large wall calendar to write down due dates and tests. Then your child can work backward to add in study days before tests and break projects down into smaller chunks.

Choose And Use A Homework Timer

Homework timers are a great way to help keep an easily distracted child on track. A timer can also give your kid a better sense of time.

There are many types of timers to choose from—what's best depends on your child. If he's distracted by sounds, a ticking kitchen timer may not be the ideal choice. Instead, try an hourglass timer or one that vibrates.

There are also homework timer apps that you can program for each subject. And don't forget that your phone probably has a timer built right in, too!

Use A Color-Coding System

Using colored dot stickers, highlighters, and colored folders and notebooks is a great (and inexpensive) way to keep organized. Ask your child to choose a color for each subject. Have him mark assignment due dates and test dates on the calendar with a sticker of the right color.

Before you file homework assignments and study guides in the appropriate notebook or folder, use a highlighter or sticker to mark the page with the right color. That way if the paper falls out, your child will know what class it's for.

Mix It Up A Little

For some kids, studying is tough because they need to learn material in different ways. If your child is having a hard time with a writing assignment, help him talk it through or act it out first. Use vocabulary words in everyday conversation—even if you have to be silly about it.

For math, use household items to help him figure out problems. Teach fractions with slices of pizza, for example. And help your child learn spelling words by letting him text them to you. You can even help him master new facts by setting them to music!

Check In And Check Up

You can't do your child's homework for him, but you can make sure he's doing it himself. Checking in to see if he needs help or just to let him know you're around may ease his homework stress. And don't forget to look over his work at the end of the day, too!

Chapter 39

Homework Strategies For Students With Learning Disabilities

> Homework can help students develop study skills that will be of value even after they leave school. It can teach them that learning takes place anywhere, not just in the classroom.
>
> *(Source: "Homework Tips For Parents," U.S. Department of Education (ED).)*

After a long day of concentration at school, settling down to homework can be difficult for any student, but it's especially challenging for teens with learning disabilities (LD). Homework is intended to reinforce classroom lessons and provide additional opportunity for learning, but often LD students experience difficulty completing homework because of such factors as attention issues, high frustration levels, forgetfulness, and trouble with organization. Just as there are special methods for helping LD students succeed in the classroom, there are strategies that can help them achieve homework goals.

Organization

The first step in getting organized to do homework actually doesn't take place at home. Before leaving class, be sure you have a clear understanding of that day's assignments. Don't be embarrassed to ask as many questions as necessary to be sure you know what has to be done. Write down the requirements, the due date, and any other pertinent details. Don't trust anything to memory. And make sure you have everything you need to complete the work, including the appropriate books, notes, and supplies.

"Homework Strategies For Students With Learning Disabilities," © 2017 Omnigraphics. Reviewed December 2016.

Timing Is Everything

It would be ideal to set aside the same time each day to begin homework. This kind of fixed schedule can help you develop good study habits, make homework a priority, and schedule other activities around your schoolwork. However, realistically, this is not always possible, since extracurricular activities, friends, and family commitments can prevent such rigid scheduling. It's a good idea to make a calendar, writing in planned activities—like sports practices and games, music lessons, and holidays—and then schedule daily homework time around them. Just be sure to allow enough time to get assignments done.

Location, Location, Location

Sure, it's possible to work on the floor in the living room or out on the patio on a nice day, but these places don't provide an ideal environment for concentration. You really need a dedicated homework space. It doesn't have to be anything fancy, but important considerations include relative quiet, few distractions, good lighting, and a comfortable chair. A desk or table with appropriate height for writing or working on a computer is also a must. And be sure your work area is stocked with all the supplies you'll need.

Have A Plan

Sometimes the number and complexity of assignments can seem overwhelming. So when you first sit down, it might help to make a checklist of tasks, in order of importance or whatever makes the most sense to you – maybe list them by due date or by difficulty. It might help to break down the most complicated assignments into smaller tasks, so they'll seem less intimidating. A list will help you get organized, keep you from forgetting anything, and give you a sense of satisfaction as you check off completed items.

Keep It Interesting

Not every homework assignment is going to be fun, but there are steps you can take to avoid that mind-numbing feeling that kills concentration. For example, you might organize your task list to alternate difficult assignments with easier ones or those you find more interesting. Take frequent breaks. After each task, listen to a song, take a walk around the house, play with a pet for a few minutes, practice a musical instrument, or watch a short video. Calling or texting a friend might provide a welcome distraction, but then you risk getting caught up in a lengthy conversation. So choose break activities wisely.

Don't Be Afraid To Ask For Help

If you get stuck or just need to bounce an idea off of someone, parents or siblings can be a valuable resource, especially if they're familiar with a topic. Some assignments lend themselves to a team approach, and in those cases, working with a classmate can be both fun and helpful. And some schools can arrange a tutor or peer support. If you feel you could use this kind of additional help, check with your guidance counselor find out what's available. Finally, after a particularly difficult assignment has been reviewed by your teacher, schedule extra time after class so you can ask for some detailed feedback and suggestions for improvement.

> Teachers assign homework for many reasons: to review what was covered in class, explore subjects more fully than classroom time allowed, extend learning by applying skills to new situations, allow students to work independently, encourage self-discipline, and teach students to use a variety of resources, such as libraries, reference materials, and the Internet.

References

1   "Five Homework Strategies for Teaching Students with Learning Disabilities," TheAllINeed.com, October 5, 2015.

2   Hutton, Lindsay. "Homework Strategies for Children with Learning Disabilities," FamilyEducation.com, n.d.

3   Morin, Amanda. "7 Tips for Improving Your Child's Homework and Study Skills," Understood.com, n.d.

4   Myers, Pam, BSEd. "Homework Strategies for Students with Learning Disabilities," Child Development Institute, May 1, 2014.

5   Warger, Cynthia. "Five Homework Strategies for Teaching Students With Learning Disabilities," LDOnline.com, 2015.

Chapter 40
Assistive Technology And Learning Disabilities

Why Using Assistive Technology For Children With Learning Disabilities

A learning disability, according to the Individuals with Disabilities Act (IDEA), is a disorder in one or more of the basic cognitive abilities involved in understanding or using spoken or written language. This could lead to an imperfect ability to listen, think, speak, read, write, spell, or do mathematical calculations. The term includes such conditions as perceptual handicaps, brain injury, minimal brain dysfunction, reading disabilities, and developmental aphasia. The term does not include children who have learning problems that are primarily the result of visual, hearing, or motor handicaps; mental retardation; emotional disturbance; or environmental, cultural, or economic disadvantage. Learning disabilities (LD) cannot be cured, but children with LD grow up with learning differences, and with persistence of proper instructions and assistive tools, they could greatly improve and attain their potentials. Such tool is assistive technology (AT).

> Assistive technology (AT) is any device that helps a learner with a disability complete an everyday task.

About This Chapter: This chapter includes text excerpted from "Using Assistive Technology In Teaching Children With Learning Disabilities In The 21st Century," Institute of Education Sciences (IES), U.S. Department of Education (ED), 2015.

AT tool is any item that is used to maintain or improve the functioning of a child with a disability. The tool can be complex (such as a complimentary communication device). The tool can be an adapted, like a tape recorder. Likewise, if one is physically handicapped, a remote control for the TV can be an AT. If someone has poor eyesight, a pair of glasses or a magnifier is an AT. The potential for AT children with LD is great, and that its benefits include enhancing academic achievement in written expression, reading, mathematics, and spelling; improving organization; and fostering social acceptance. It was viewed that support (assistive) technology provides many benefits by facilitating writing for children with LD who often find the writing process frustrating. It therefore means that when children have the chance to accommodate writing challenges, they are more excellent in the classroom. An essential element of this attempt is partnership between classroom teachers and AT specialists. The use of AT must be a joint effort.

To achieve this laudable feat in improving the learning of children with LD, principles behind the introduction of this technology into the teaching-learning process were identified:

- AT can only enhance basic skills, and not replacing them. It should be used as part of the educational process, and can be used to teach basic skills.

- AT for children with disabilities is more than an educational tool; it is a fundamental work tool that is comparable to pencil and paper for non-disabled children.

- Children with disabilities use AT to access and use standard tools, complete educational tasks, and participate on an equal basis with their developing peers in the regular educational environment.

- The use of AT does not automatically make educational and commercial software/tools accessible or usable.

- An AT evaluation conducted by a professional, knowledgeable in regular and AT, is needed to determine whether a child requires AT devices and services and should be specified in the children's instructional plans.

- AT evaluation must address the alternative and augmentative communication needs, that is, ability to communicate needs and change the environment for children with disabilities.

- To be effective, an AT evaluation should be ongoing process.

It was maintained that sticking to these principles, AT assists to enhance the independence of children with LD, because oftentimes, these children bank on parents, siblings, friends and teachers for assistance. Relying on others may slow the transition into adulthood, and may also lower self-esteem, as it demands children with LD to depend on others, rather than themselves, to solve a problem. AT moreover, provides a way for children with LD to achieve specific tasks on their own.

Various Types Of Assistive Technology For Children With Learning Disabilities

AT is capable of addressing many types of learning difficulties. It was stated that a child who has difficulty writing can compose a school report by dictating it and having it converted to text by special software. Moreso, a child who struggles with arithmetic problem can use a hand-held calculator to keep score while playing a game with a friend. Also, a teenager with dyslexia may benefit from AT that will read aloud from the textbook guide. A child who cannot speak may need a communication device such as a language board or a device with a speech synthesizer to participate in class. Additionally, a child with a learning disability may need a computer programmes to learn to read. AT has usually been applied to computer hardware and software and electronic tools. The AT tools help children with LD, who struggle with listening, mathematics, organization and memory, reading and writing skills. Each of the skills is listed and how AT could help to solve the learning skills.

Written Language Assistive Technologies

Some of the written language AT tools that help children with LD include:

- **Spell Checkers:** They are part of word processing programmes with vary sizes which could be portable or stationed. They could be attached to word processors to scan written documents and display to the user or children the misspelled words and speak the words by ways of speech synthesizer. The disadvantage of these tools is that when two words sound the same (there, their), the child find it difficult to choose the correct word suitable for the sentence, as the tool do not recognize and offer suggestions for correct spellings.

- **Proofreading:** otherwise called "grammar checkers." They check for errors in grammar, capitalization, and word usage. The errors are identified on the computer screen and the child corrects.

- **Speech Synthesizers:** These tools give the children the opportunity to hear spoken text on the computer monitor. The child can review the text already written down and read it from the monitor and at the same time hears the spoken words from the computer. This is to enable the child to know if the text he or she writes down makes sense. These tools allow children to spell words and hear them pronounced correctly rather than phonetically.

- **Speech Recognition:** This system allows the child to speak to the computer through a microphone, and the spoken words show as texts on the computer monitor. If this system recognizes words incorrectly, the child can have the opportunity to choose from the list of similar sounding words shown on the monitor. The speech recognition tool is most useful to children who have better oral language abilities than written language.

Reading Assistive Technologies

Some of the reading AT tools that help children with LD includes:

- **Microsoft Word:** One of the easiest differentiation tools for a reading passage is a software programme that most teachers have readily at hand—Microsoft Word. Smaller reading passages copied and pasted into Microsoft Word, can be easily enhanced to aid comprehension using standard formatting features within the programme. Using the highlighting feature can help students focus on particular aspects of a text like parts of speech, literary devices, or key elements of a paragraph.

- **Tape Recorders:** These tools are used to play audio taped text by children with reading disabilities. The child listens to the recorded texts in books or printed materials rather than reading it.

- **Speech Synthesis:** This tool can serve the purpose of reading engine. It could be available on computer disc loaded to the computer and then the child read back by the speech synthesizer.

- **Optical Character Recognition (OCR):** This tool could be connected with speech synthesis. It enables the child to type printed text to the computer, while the speech synthesizer reads the text back and aloud for the child to hear and alongside see the text. This device also works with scanner that reads images and text from the written or printed materials. Texts or words are inputted data into the computer file shown on the screen, and thereafter change the printed text from the scanner to computer text. This tool therefore is useful for children with reading disabilities to read printed words, and also those children who understand better what they hear than what they could see. Also, the software makes the resulting computer file capable of being edited.

- **Variable Speech Control (VSC):** This tool is in form of tape recorder, which enable the child to play the texts recorded in audio tape very fast than the originally recorded, with all the sounds of the words still intact. This is very useful for children who better understand when texts are presented at a slow rate.

Mathematics Assistive Technologies

Some of the mathematics AT tools that help children with LD includes:

- **Electronic Mathematics Worksheets:** These worksheets could assist children with arithmetic problems to arrange, ally and route through the basic mathematical sums with the use of a computer. The basic mathematical problem like addition, subtraction, division and multiplication are inputted into the computer through keyboard or mouse. The tool will automatically align itself to correct vertical format. The inputted numbers will be read aloud by the child through the use of speech synthesizer. This is beneficial to children with arithmetic problems, in that, it helps to align or arrange math problems with pencil and paper.

- **Talking Calculators:** This tool is used to speak a number, symbols, and other operation keys, with the use of speech synthesizer, whenever a child presses the keys. When completed, the child could read back the answers from the completed calculations. By listening to it, the child could find the inputted errors, when wrong keys are pressed. It could also help the child to double check for errors, when copying numbers or symbols.

Listening Assistive Technologies

Some of the listening AT tools that help children with LD includes:

- **FM Listening Systems:** These tools are used with the help of a small-sized transmitter unit, together with the microphone. The tool redirects child's voice straight to his or her ear. This makes the child/speaker's voice louder. The advantage of these tools to the children with listening problem is, it enables them to hear what the teacher or the speaker is saying.

- **Tape Recorders:** These tools are used by children with listening problems to capture spoke information of the speaker or teacher's lesson. These recorders allow children to the oral presentation again and again, especially for those children who have problems processing, understanding or remembering what they hear.

Memory/Organization Assistive Technologies

Some of the listening AT tools that help children with LD includes:

- **Personal Data Managers:** These data managers could be in form of software packages, which could be used for a computer or as electronic devices. They are useful for children with memory or organizational problems to store and retrieve large information from the system, as in saving phone numbers, keeping memorable dates and appointments; forming a reminder for the users.

- **Free-form databases:** These databases allow children with memory problems to type or enter notes or pieces of information into the computer, rather than or as written down in a piece of paper. The child can retrieve the information from the screen of the computer whenever he or she needs them, and serve as reminders to the child.

- **Prewriting organizers:** The writing process involves a number of stages. Many children have difficulty with the preparation stage, which integrates brainstorming, clustering, and listing ideas, themes, or keywords. Some children with memory problems find graphic organizers helpful in mapping ideas during the planning stage. Graphic organizers such as Inspiration provide organizational frameworks to help children generate topics and content for writing projects. Inspiration shows ideas in graphic "bubbles" that can be moved and then converted into a standard outline.

Choosing The Right Technology For Children With Learning Disabilities

In today's learning environments, a wide range of technologies is creating new alternatives for differentiating instruction and supporting the contribution of children with LD. With an array of AT available in the stores and on the Internet for teachers and parents to select, there is no fast rule in choosing the right ones for children with LD.

Nevertheless, the choice of the appropriate use of AT, whether available or improvised, the right selection depends on the individual child, the skills problems, the setting and the particular tasks the child wants to achieve. This implies that one tool used for a child may not be useful for another child in a different setting. Some of the guidelines that may assist children with learning disabilities achieve amidst the array of ATs are discussed below:

Determine The Child's Specific Problem

The use of AT tools should depend on the identified problems of the child with LD. For instance, AT could help solve the problem of writing difficulty, such as problems with grammar or compensate for a memory problem should be selected to meet or support the child's specific problems.

Identify The Child's Strengths

AT could work best when it is used to develop the potential of children with LD. For instance, a child who has problem reading printed words, other than who easily understands spoken words, might benefit from an optical character recognition (OCR) / speech synthesis system that changes printed words to computerized speech.

Involve The Child In The Selection Process

The interest of the child in the AT tools is paramount to the selection of the tools. This will enable the child to easily learn how to use the tools that will translate to change in the teaching-learning process. The parents or teachers should therefore consider this in the selection and purchase of tools, as well as in the developing the child's interest in the tools.

Choose The Types Of Technology That Are Helpful And Based On The Child's Strengths And Weaknesses

Always consider that the technologies that are useful to your child's needs are important to him or her, than just purchasing and using the ones that would not meet the identified needs or problems. Technology can be quite impressive, with all its shapes and designs, but not necessarily helpful to the child.

Determine The Specific Settings For The Technology

The location of the technology for the child could be at home, school, playing ground, open space or in a social setting. Placing the one that supposed to be used at home, in the school could be a wrong choice, and would not serve the right purpose for the child. The setting for the technology could include where they could be stored or kept and the right furniture to place them.

Choose Technologies That Work Together

Imagine a speech recognition system that would not work or incompatible with the current computer window system could pose a problem and could be frustrating.

Choose Technologies That Are Easy To Learn And Operate

Consider a child or learner with LD that has difficulties in memory and other cognitive problems, finding it difficult to use and operate most of the ATs; this may not benefit them if they found it hard to manipulate the tools. They may as well lose interest in such tools.

Therefore, choosing the easy-to-operate devices will be helpful and develop an interest in the child.

Instructional Guidelines For The Teachers

For children with LD to benefit maximally from the use of AT tools, whether in the classroom or at home, teacher should follow some basic guidelines that will enable the use of AT worthwhile and making the teaching-learning process enjoyable and productive. The following basic guidelines should be followed and adhered to by the classroom teachers:

- Teachers should know that every child's AT needs are distinctive. Children's needs should be matched with necessary technology rather than matching available tools to student needs.

- Teachers should teach needed technology skills before they are required. Thus, the children can then pay attention on regular classroom instruction rather than simultaneously learning the curriculum and the new AT skills.

- It is very important that technology training for teachers make children better users of AT and maximizes the impact of efforts and finances expended. Teachers should be up-to-date in the AT skills acquisition. This training should include making teachers spend time researching and reading the recommended books and be current in the global use of ATs.

- It is also important that teachers should have access to technical supports that might help in case of any system's crash or breakdown.

- The global trend now is collaboration and partnership among the multidisciplinary team that may include AT teacher, computer teacher, and computer maintenance professionals. This will help to ensure a functional/faultless AT environment.

Chapter 41

Testing Accommodation For Students With Disabilities

Standardized examinations and other high-stakes tests are gateways to educational and employment opportunities. Whether seeking admission to a high school, college, or graduate program, or attempting to obtain a professional license or certification for a trade, it is difficult to achieve such goals without sitting for some kind of standardized exam or high-stakes test.

The Americans with Disabilities Act (ADA) ensures that individuals with disabilities have the opportunity to fairly compete for and pursue such opportunities by requiring testing entities to offer exams in a manner accessible to persons with disabilities. When needed testing accommodations are provided, test-takers can demonstrate their true aptitude.

What Kinds Of Tests Are Covered?

Exams administered by any private, state, or local government entity related to applications, licensing, certification, or credentialing for secondary or postsecondary education, professional, or trade purposes are covered by the ADA and testing accommodations, pursuant to the ADA, must be provided.

Examples of covered exams include:

- high school equivalency exams (such as the GED);

- high school entrance exams (such as the SSAT or ISEE);

- college entrance exams (such as the SAT or ACT);

- exams for admission to professional schools (such as the LSAT or MCAT);

About This Chapter: This chapter includes text excerpted from "ADA Requirements: Testing Accommodations," Americans with Disabilities Act (ADA), U.S. Department of Justice (DOJ), 2014.

- admissions exams for graduate schools (such as the GRE or GMAT); and

- licensing exams for trade purposes (such as cosmetology) or professional purposes (such as bar exams or medical licensing exams, including clinical assessments).

What Are Testing Accommodations?

Testing accommodations are changes to the regular testing environment and auxiliary aids and services that allow individuals with disabilities to demonstrate their true aptitude or achievement level on standardized exams or other high-stakes tests.

Examples of the wide range of testing accommodations that may be required include:

- Braille or large-print exam booklets;

- screen reading technology;

- scribes to transfer answers to Scantron bubble sheets or record dictated notes and essays;

- extended time;

- wheelchair-accessible testing stations;

- distraction-free rooms;

- physical prompts (such as for individuals with hearing impairments); and

- permission to bring and take medications during the exam (for example, for individuals with diabetes who must monitor their blood sugar and administer insulin).

Who Is Eligible To Receive Testing Accommodations?

Individuals with disabilities are eligible to receive necessary testing accommodations. Under the ADA, an individual with a disability is a person who has a physical or mental impairment that substantially limits a major life activity (such as seeing, hearing, learning, reading, concentrating, or thinking) or a major bodily function (such as the neurological, endocrine, or digestive system). The determination of whether an individual has a disability generally should not demand extensive analysis and must be made without regard to any positive effects of measures such as medication, medical supplies or equipment, low-vision devices (other than ordinary eyeglasses or contact lenses), prosthetics, hearing aids and cochlear implants, or mobility devices. However, negative effects, such as side effects of medication or burdens associated with following a particular treatment regimen, may be considered when determining whether an individual's impairment substantially limits a major life activity.

A person with a history of academic success may still be a person with a disability who is entitled to testing accommodations under the ADA. A history of academic success does not mean that a person does not have a disability that requires testing accommodations. For example, someone with a learning disability may achieve a high level of academic success, but may nevertheless be substantially limited in one or more of the major life activities of reading, writing, speaking, or learning, because of the additional time or effort he or she must spend to read, write, speak, or learn compared to most people in the general population.

What Testing Accommodations Must Be Provided?

Testing entities must ensure that the test scores of individuals with disabilities accurately reflect the individual's aptitude or achievement level or whatever skill the exam or test is intended to measure. A testing entity must administer its exam so that it accurately reflects an individual's aptitude, achievement level, or the skill that the exam purports to measure, rather than the individual's impairment (except where the impaired skill is one the exam purports to measure).

Example: An individual may be entitled to the use of a basic calculator during exams as a testing accommodation. If the objective of the test is to measure one's ability to solve algebra equations, for example, and the ability to perform basic math computations (e.g., addition, subtraction, multiplication, and division), is secondary to the objective of the test, then a basic calculator may be an appropriate testing accommodation. If, however, the objective of the test is to measure the individual's understanding of, and ability to perform, math computations, then it likely would not be appropriate to permit a calculator as a testing accommodation.

What Kind Of Documentation Is Sufficient To Support A Request For Testing Accommodations?

All testing entities must adhere to the following principles regarding what may and may not be required when a person with a disability requests a testing accommodation.

Documentation. Any documentation if required by a testing entity in support of a request for testing accommodations must be reasonable and limited to the need for the requested testing accommodations. Requests for supporting documentation should be narrowly tailored to the information needed to determine the nature of the candidate's disability and his or her need for the requested testing accommodation. Appropriate documentation will vary depending on the nature of the disability and the specific testing accommodation requested.

Examples of types of documentation include:

- recommendations of qualified professionals;

- proof of past testing accommodations;

- observations by educators;

- results of psycho-educational or other professional evaluations;

- an applicant's history of diagnosis; and

- an applicant's statement of his or her history regarding testing accommodations.

Depending on the particular testing accommodation request and the nature of the disability, however, a testing entity may only need one or two of the above documents to determine the nature of the candidate's disability and his or her need for the requested testing accommodation. If so, a testing entity should generally limit its request for documentation to those one or two items and should generally evaluate the testing accommodation request based on those limited documents without requiring further documentation.

- **Past testing accommodations.** Proof of past testing accommodations in similar test settings is generally sufficient to support a request for the same testing accommodations for a current standardized exam or other high-stakes test.

- **Formal public school accommodations.** If a candidate previously received testing accommodations under an Individualized Education Program (IEP) or a Section 504 Plan, he or she should generally receive the same testing accommodations for a current standardized exam or high-stakes test.

- **Private school testing accommodations.** If a candidate received testing accommodations in private school for similar tests under a formal policy, he or she should generally receive the same testing accommodations for a current standardized exam or high-stakes test.

- **First time requests or informal classroom testing accommodations.** An absence of previous formal testing accommodations does not preclude a candidate from receiving testing accommodations.

- **Qualified professionals.** Testing entities should defer to documentation from a qualified professional who has made an individualized assessment of the candidate that supports the need for the requested testing accommodations.

How Quickly Should A Testing Entity Respond To A Request For Testing Accommodations?

A testing entity must respond in a timely manner to requests for testing accommodations so as to ensure equal opportunity for individuals with disabilities. Testing entities should ensure that their process for reviewing and approving testing accommodations responds in time for applicants to register and prepare for the test. In addition, the process should provide applicants with a reasonable opportunity to respond to any requests for additional information from the testing entity, and still be able to take the test in the same testing cycle. Failure by a testing entity to act in a timely manner, coupled with seeking unnecessary documentation, could result in such an extended delay that it constitutes a denial of equal opportunity or equal treatment in an examination setting for persons with disabilities.

How Should Testing Entities Report Test Scores For Test-Takers Receiving Disability-Related Accommodations?

Testing entities should report accommodated scores in the same way they report scores generally. Testing entities must not decline to report scores for test-takers with disabilities receiving accommodations under the ADA.

Flagging policies that impede individuals with disabilities from fairly competing for and pursuing educational and employment opportunities are prohibited by the ADA. "Flagging" is the policy of annotating test scores or otherwise reporting scores in a manner that indicates the exam was taken with a testing accommodation. Flagging announces to anyone receiving the exam scores that the test-taker has a disability and suggests that the scores are not valid or deserved. Flagging also discourages test-takers with disabilities from exercising their right to testing accommodations under the ADA for fear of discrimination. Flagging must not be used to circumvent the requirement that testing entities provide testing accommodations for persons with disabilities and ensure that the test results for persons with disabilities reflect their abilities, not their disabilities.

233

Chapter 42

Educational Options After High School

Students with learning disabilities (LD) have many options for continuing their education after high school, including four-year universities, two-year colleges, vocational or technical programs, adult basic education (ABE) or continuing education programs, and life skills training. The unique challenges of LD make it especially important for you to plan ahead, set goals, and stay organized as you consider your postsecondary education options. Planning for college can begin as early as your freshman year of high school. You should work with your teachers, guidance counselors, and Individual Education Plan (IEP) team to select courses that will help prepare you for success in college and in your transition to adulthood.

Planning For College

The process of planning for postsecondary education includes the following steps:

- **Identify your interests**

    High school is an ideal time to identify your personal interests and explore possible career paths in those areas. School guidance counselors can provide you with various tools and assessments to help you find career options that fit your strengths and interests. You can also learn about potential careers by attending job fairs, talking with people who work in fields of interest to you, and volunteering or job shadowing.

"Educational Options After High School," © 2017 Omnigraphics. Reviewed January 2017.

- **Practice self-advocacy**

  Self-advocacy means speaking up for yourself and taking more responsibility for the decisions affecting your life. Practicing self-advocacy in high school helps you gain the independence you will need in college. You can become a stronger self-advocate by understanding your disability and how it impacts your learning, and by asking for accommodations in a positive way. Once you reach college, these skills will help you take responsibility for planning your future and accessing the support services you need to get there.

- **Improve your study habits**

  Your success in college will depend on your ability to stay organized and use your time wisely. You will need to take responsibility for managing your class schedule, doing your homework, and using the study methods that work best for you. Working to develop strong study habits in high school gives you an advantage in making the transition to college.

- **Prepare for college entrance exams**

  Students with LD are eligible for test-taking accommodations on the ACT and SAT college entrance exams. These tests are typically taken in the spring of your junior year of high school and in the fall of your senior year of high school. A variety of online and community resources are available to help students prepare and practice for these standardized tests.

- **Research schools and programs**

  Your high school guidance counselor can provide a vast amount of information about postsecondary educational options. The key is to identify the schools and programs that best match your career interests and your academic abilities. Research the requirements for admission and graduation to see whether you meet them. You can also contact the disability services offices at various schools to inquire about the supports and accommodations they offer for students with LD.

Did you know...

According to a 2014 survey by the National Center for Learning Disabilities, 54 percent of high school students with LD planned to attend a two-year or four-year college, while 43 percent planned to pursue vocational or technical training.

Postsecondary Educational Options

Once you narrow down your career interests and future goals, you are ready to decide which type of postsecondary education option best fits your needs. The main choices include the following:

- **Four-year colleges and universities**

  There are nearly 2,500 of these institutions in the United States. They can be public or private, and they vary by size, courses of study offered, admission requirements, and academic standards. Students who complete a degree program typically earn a bachelor's degree. Those who are interested in careers that require advanced training may also attend graduate or professional schools to earn a master's or doctoral degree.

- **Two-year community or junior colleges**

  There are more than 1,000 of these institutions in the United States. Although they vary in size and can be public or private, most have easier admissions policies than larger universities and also tend to be less expensive. Students who complete a degree program typically earn an associate's or applied science degree. Some two-year degree programs prepare you for specific careers—such as accounting or criminal justice—while others allow you to earn credits that will transfer to a four-year college. Most public community colleges do not offer student housing, so they tend to serve people from the local community.

- **Vocational and technical schools**

  These programs offer specialized training to prepare students for particular occupations, such as computer technician, plumber, broadcast technician, medical assistant, veterinary assistant, truck driver, or cosmetologist. They may be public or private.

- **Adult and continuing education programs**

  Adult Basic Education (ABE) programs offer free tutoring and instruction in basic skills like reading, writing, and math for students who have not yet earned a high school diploma. Students can improve their literacy and academic skills in order to take the high-school equivalency exam. Continuing education classes can be found at many community colleges and some four-year universities. These courses have minimal admission standards and offer training in a variety of fields, such as marketing, technology, food management, and health services. Some students take continuing education courses to explore their personal interests, while others receive certification in specific fields.

- **Life skills training**

    These programs offer training in social skills, life management skills, and independent living for students who may not be able to attend college or vocational programs.

In order to choose the best postsecondary educational option for you, it is important to investigate the level of support available for students with LD in each setting. Since the It is a good idea to visit campuses, meet with representatives from the office of disability support services, and inquire whether the school or program will provide accommodations that meet your needs.

References

1. "At a Glance: Types of Colleges and How They Differ," Understood, 2016.

2. "Information for Students with Disabilities," EducationQuest.

3. "Post-Secondary Educational Options," Learning Disabilities Association of America, 2017.

4. Stefanakos, Victoria Scanlan. "Planning for College: A Four-Year Guide for High School Students," Understood, 2016.

Chapter 43
Transition Planning

What Is Transition?

The transition from youth to adulthood is critical for every young person. This is particularly true for young people with disabilities. Ideally, during the transition years, youth acquire knowledge and learn important skills they will need to maximize their independence and self-sufficiency in their communities. This process involves multiple domains including community engagement, education, employment, health, and independent living. It includes accessing educational opportunities including vocational training, obtaining employment, finding stable housing, and accessing healthcare and other resources to support their future planning and development into adulthood.

> Transition is the period of time when adolescents are moving into adulthood and are often concerned with planning for postsecondary education, careers, healthcare, financial benefits, housing, and more. Research shows that regardless of eligibility and access challenges, there is a need to provide continuity of service for youth from ages 14 or 16 to ages 25 or 30 across child- and adult-service systems.

About This Chapter: Text under the heading "What Is Transition?" is excerpted from "The 2020 Federal Youth Transition Plan: A Federal Interagency Strategy," Federal Partners in Transition (FPT), February 2015; Text under the heading "What Is Transition Planning?" is excerpted from "What Is Transition Planning?" Disability.gov, U.S. Department of Labor (DOL), April 18, 2014.

What Is Transition Planning?

The National Collaborative on Workforce and Development (NCWD) for Youth defines transition planning as:

"…a coordinated set of activities for a student with a disability that: A) Is designed within an outcome-oriented process, that promotes movement from school-to-post-school activities, including postsecondary education, vocational training, integrated employment (including supported employment), continuing and adult education, adult services, independent living, or community participation; B) Is based upon the individual student's needs, taking into account the student's preferences and interests; and C) Includes instruction, related services, special education, community experiences, the development of employment and other post-school adult living objectives, and when appropriate, the acquisition of daily living skills and functional vocational evaluation."

The transition planning process should begin around middle school and continue throughout high school. The student, his or her parents or guardians, teachers and school counselors should work together to develop a plan for life after high school. This plan should take into account the student's strengths, preferences, and interests, as well as any accommodations needs and other key factors. The types of questions to think about are similar to what any student would need to address, with a few additional considerations:

- What types of things interest this student? Is he or she creative and thinking about going into the arts? Is there an interest in a particular field, such as journalism or mathematics?

- Is the student thinking about going to college? If so, which type of school would be a good fit (community college, in-state four-year university, out-of-state university, etc.)?

- Is the student thinking about training for a trade? If so, what schools or programs are available? Which would be a good fit for him/her?

- Which standardized tests does the student need to take to apply for colleges or technical/trade schools? Will the student need any accommodations while taking these tests?

- What types of accommodations would the student need in college or at technical/trade school?

- What are the student's financial needs? Does he or she want to apply for student aid? Which types of aid would be best (e.g., loans, grants, scholarships)? When are the applications due? What information needs to be provided?

- Which type of living situation is the student interested in (e.g., at home, college dorm, on his/her own) and what types of accommodations will the student need?

- Is the student interested in going directly into the workforce? What job training, internship or apprenticeship opportunities are available?

Ideally, the transition planning process should involve students, parents, teachers and guidance counselors (or other education professionals) discussing what they hope for after high school.

Chapter 44

Career Preparation And Work-Based Learning Experiences

Career preparation and work-based learning experiences are essential in order to form and develop aspirations and to make informed choices about careers. These experiences can be provided during the school day, or through after-school programs, and will require collaborations with other organizations. All youth need information on career options, including:

- career assessments to help identify students' school and post-school preferences and interests

- structured exposure to postsecondary education and other lifelong learning opportunities

- exposure to career opportunities that ultimately lead to a living wage, including information about educational requirements, entry requirements, income and benefits potential, and asset accumulation, and

- training designed to improve job-seeking skills and workplace basic skills (sometimes called soft skills).

In order to identify and attain career goals, youth need to be exposed to a range of experiences, including:

- opportunities to engage in a range of work-based exploration activities such as site visits and job shadowing

About This Chapter: Text in this chapter begins with excerpts from "Youth In Transition: Career Preparation And Work-Based Learning Experiences," U.S. Department of Labor (DOL), August 3, 2011. Reviewed December 2016; Text beginning with the heading "Work-Based Learning Experiences—Why They Are Important" is excerpted from "Pathway To Employment For Youth With Disabilities," Corporation for National and Community Service, Office of Disability Employment Policy (ODEP), U.S. Department of Labor (DOL), June 15, 2013. Reviewed December 2016.

- multiple on-the-job training experiences, including community service (paid or unpaid) that is specifically linked to the content of a program of study and school credit

- opportunities to learn and practice their work skills ("soft skills"), and

- opportunities to learn first-hand about specific occupational skills related to a career pathway.

In addition, youth with disabilities need to:

- understand the relationships between benefits planning and career choices

- learn to communicate their disability-related work support and accommodation needs

- learn to find, formally request and secure appropriate supports and reasonable accommodations in education, training, and employment settings

Work-Based Learning Experiences—Why They Are Important

Work experiences, both paid and voluntary, have been recognized as critical components of preparing youth, including those with disabilities, for the transition to adulthood. Volunteerism and service-learning are included among these on-the-job training experiences that can help prepare youth by:

- developing career readiness skills, including basic work skills (or "soft skills"), such as attendance, punctuality, teamwork, and conflict resolution;

- providing knowledge of specific occupational skills;

- offering opportunities to establish a work history and connections; and

- providing a forum for exploring different occupations.

Even short-term work experiences can be valuable as a way for all youth to develop skills, contacts, and awareness about career options. Research shows that having a competitive paid job in secondary school is the strongest predictor of job success for youth with disabilities after graduation. Moreover, both paid and unpaid work experiences help youth with disabilities acquire jobs at higher wages after they graduate.

Benefits Associated With Service Learning And Volunteerism

Numerous studies have identified that youth who participate in quality community-based service-learning experiences can gain the following benefits and others which contribute to improved transition outcomes and positive youth development:

- access to the range of supports and opportunities (or developmental assets) they need to grow up healthy, caring, and responsible

- increased civic engagement and community involvement

- improved understanding of how they can impact social challenges

- higher academic achievement and interest in furthering their education

- enhanced problem-solving skills, ability to work in teams, and planning abilities

For youth with disabilities, service learning provides an additional benefit. By being actively engaged in service to their communities, they gain a sense of increased self-worth associated with being providers rather than service recipients.

The Link Between Volunteerism And Competitive Employment

The Corporation for National and Community Service (CNCS) is an independent federal agency with the responsibility to mobilize Americans into service through three programs: Senior Corps, AmeriCorps, and The Social innovation Fund. These programs support service-learning in schools, higher education institutions, community-based organizations, and full-time service across the nation.

A research released by CNCS in June 2013 provides the most compelling empirical research to date establishing an association between volunteering and employment in the United States. Key findings on the connection between volunteering and employment include the following:

- Volunteers have a 27 percent higher likelihood of finding a job after being out of work than non-volunteers;

- Volunteers without a high school diploma have a 51 percent higher likelihood of finding employment;

- Volunteers living in rural areas have a 55 percent higher likelihood of finding employment.

CNCS also found that volunteering is associated with an increased likelihood of finding employment for all volunteers regardless of a person's gender, age, ethnicity, geographical area, or the job market conditions.

According to CNCS, volunteering can help people find employment because:

- Volunteering increases an individual's networks and connections;

- Volunteering increases an individual's experience or useful education, skills, and training; and,

- Volunteering helps to create a positive impression in a competitive job market.

Part Six
Living With A Learning Disability

Chapter 45
Self-Esteem Issues And Children With Learning Disabilities

Self-esteem refers to positive feelings of worth, acceptance, and value that people hold with regard to themselves. Children who have high self-esteem feel proud, confident, secure, and capable. These feelings enable them to act independently, take responsibility for their actions, stand up for themselves, and face challenges. They are more likely to be resilient and keep trying if they make a mistake, and to have the courage to make good decisions in the face of peer pressure. Children with low self-esteem, on the other hand, lack confidence and do not believe they have value and are worthy of respect. They are less likely to stand up for themselves or ask for help, and they are more likely to give in to peer pressure.

How Self-Esteem Develops

Self-esteem begins to develop in infancy. In childhood, when the primary influences are loving parents, most people have very positive self-esteem. Toddlers, for instance, often respond with enthusiasm when asked if they are smart or able to do something. Young children try new things, experience repeated successes, and receive praise for their efforts. This pattern gives them confidence to face additional challenges and makes them feel good about themselves. Over time, they develop the positive characteristics associated with high self-esteem.

As children reach school age, however, they gradually begin incorporating more negative feedback from the classroom and other parts of the outside world. They experience failures, and their efforts are not always rewarded. Around the age of seven, children begin comparing themselves to their peers and realizing that others may possess stronger skills in some areas. As a result, their confidence and self-esteem may begin to wane.

"Self-Esteem Issues And Children With Learning Disabilities," © 2017 Omnigraphics. Reviewed June 2016.

Learning Disabilities And Self-Esteem

This process affects children with learning disabilities to a greater degree than most other children. Children with learning disabilities tend to experience more failure and receive more negative feedback. They also compare themselves unfavorably to their peers in terms of academic skills and performance. Schoolwork comes less easily to them and can sometimes seem impossible. Although many children with learning disabilities or attention issues are accepted by their peers, some become targets of teasing or bullying.

As a result, research suggests that children with learning disabilities tend to have lower self-esteem than their peers. After years of academic struggles and frustration, they often view themselves as being "stupid" or "slow" in comparison with other children. They tend to generalize these feelings and perceive themselves negatively in other areas of life as well. Due to low self-esteem, children with learning disabilities may lose interest in learning, develop self-defeating ways of dealing with challenges, and perform poorly, which only reinforces their low self-worth.

Ways Parents Can Impact Self-Esteem

Fortunately, parents, siblings, friends, teachers, and other influential people can help bolster children's self-esteem. Experts stress that it is possible for children to learn to improve the way they view themselves and their abilities. For parents of children with learning disabilities, being supportive yet realistic is the key to helping children build their self-esteem. While praise and positive feedback is important, it becomes meaningless if it is offered insincerely. When parents lavish praise on everything a child does, the child may begin to distrust it or overreact to negative feedback. Parents can incorporate the following suggestions to help children with learning disabilities develop higher self-esteem:

- Emphasize that the child is bright and healthy, and that they just have a deficit in a certain area of learning.

- Encourage the child's non-academic interests—such as art, music, or sports—and highlight their areas of strength—such as kindness or a sense of humor.

- Provide an example of how to value personal strengths while also acknowledging and working to improve upon weaknesses.

- Offer examples of successful people who have overcome learning disabilities and achieved their dreams.

- Express clear, realistic expectations instead of criticisms. For instance, instead of complaining that the child's room is always messy, ask the child to put away their toys and make their bed.

- Ensure that the child has plenty of opportunities to be successful.

- Help the child view mistakes as learning experiences for next time.

- Avoid comparing the child to other people—such as siblings or classmates—and only evaluate their performance in relation to previous efforts.

- Help the child develop positive strategies for learning and coping with challenges.

- Help the child build effective problem-solving and decision-making skills. Rather than providing solutions, help them brainstorm creative approaches and consider the possible consequences of each one.

- Teach the child to reframe negative statements.

- Help the child find friends who accept them and make them feel valued.

- Encourage the child to help others by volunteering in the community. Having something valuable to offer to other people bolsters self-esteem.

- Provide a safe haven where the child feels loved, appreciated, and supported. Studies show that children who are made to feel special by an adult develop increased hopefulness and resilience.

Self-esteem is a tremendous asset to help children manage learning disabilities successfully. Parents can play an important role in building self-confidence and empowering children with learning disabilities to overcome the challenges they face.

References

1. Cunningham, Bob. "The Importance of Self-Esteem for Kids with Learning and Attention Issues," Understood, 2016.

2. Lyons, Aoife. "Self-Esteem and Learning Disabilities," Learning Disabilities Association of Illinois, 2012.

3. Tracey, Danielle. "Self-Esteem and Children's Learning Problems," Learning Links, November 2012.

Chapter 46
Self-Advocacy For Students With Learning Disabilities

Speaking up for yourself is never easy. It is common to feel nervous or embarrassed when you have to approach a teacher to ask for extra time to complete an assignment, for instance, or tell a classmate that they are doing something that bothers you. The ability to express your feelings, ask for what you want, and promote your own interests is called self-advocacy. It is a valuable skill to learn—especially for teens with learning disabilities. Becoming a self-advocate means playing a more active role in decisions that affect your life. Self-advocacy empowers you to take greater control over situations you face at school, at work, or in the community. For teens with learning disabilities, self-advocacy also involves understanding your rights, requesting accommodations, and accessing the services and supports you need to be successful.

How To Become A Self-Advocate

Up to now, adults may have stepped in to advocate for you in educational or social settings. As you transition to adulthood, however, you will need to take greater responsibility for protecting your own rights and interests. Luckily, it is possible to develop or strengthen self-advocacy skills. Here are some tips for learning to be an effective self-advocate:

- **Know yourself**

  Before you can speak up for yourself, you need to understand what you want and need. After all, learning strategies and accommodations that work for one student may not be the best ones for you. Thinking about your strengths and weaknesses, and the tools and strategies that best complement your learning style, allows you to be specific in asking for help.

"Self-Advocacy For Students With Learning Disabilities," © 2017 Omnigraphics. Reviewed January 2017.

- **Know your rights**

  If you have a diagnosed learning disability, you have the legal right to reasonable accommodations at school or at work. In order to self-advocate for those rights, however, you need to understand exactly what they are. Learn how disability law applies to your situation and know the details of your Individualized Education Plan (IEP). This way, you will be well-equipped to play a bigger role in your own educational decisions.

- **Practice speaking up**

  Once you understand your personal needs and your rights under the law, you are ready to begin speaking up. You could start by sharing your thoughts and opinions in everyday situations. Some examples include raising your hand in class or joining a family discussion at the dinner table. Next, you could try asking questions to clarify what your teacher, counselor, or doctor says. As you begin to gain confidence, you can expand your self-advocacy to include asking for accommodations or standing up for your rights.

  If self-advocacy makes you feel nervous, you might find it helpful to practice what you want to say ahead of time. You could write down your main points and say them out loud to a trusted friend or to yourself in front of the mirror. Your goals should be to strike a balance between being assertive and being respectful. Other people will be more likely to listen to your concerns and try to help you if you approach them as problem-solving partners rather than adversaries.

- **Build a supportive team**

  Self-advocacy becomes much easier when you have a team of supportive people on your side. People you know and trust—including friends, family members, teachers, academic advisors, doctors, counselors, coaches, and religious leaders—are usually eager to help you become a strong self-advocate. You may also gain confidence and feel more comfortable asking for accommodations by speaking with fellow students who receive support for learning disabilities. Forming a community of self-advocates can help everyone achieve their common goals.

Did You Know...

A great way to improve your self-advocacy skills is by attending your Individualized Education Program (IEP) meetings. Federal law says you must be invited to these meetings once you reach the age of sixteen. Working with your IEP team, you can practice explaining your disability, setting educational goals, and asking for accommodations in a supportive setting.

Although self-advocacy may feel awkward or scary, it is important to remember that you have the right to ask for the resources you need to be happy and successful. You should not feel embarrassed about needing help, and you should not give up if you run into obstacles. Self-advocacy is a skill that you can learn, practice, and improve over time. Mastering it will give you the power to make choices and determine the course of your own life.

References

1. McLelland, Corrin. "Self-Advocacy," Disability Rights UK, April 20, 2015.

2. Weigel, Dessie. "Self-Advocacy: Five Tips from a Student," National Center for Learning Disabilities (NCLD), 2017.

3. "Youth in Action! Becoming a Stronger Self-Advocate," National Collaborative on Workforce and Disability for Youth (NCWD/Youth), 2015.

Chapter 47

Overcoming Common Disability Barriers

Nearly everyone faces hardships and difficulties at one time or another. But for people with disabilities, barriers can be more frequent and have greater impact. The World Health Organization (WHO) describes barriers as being more than just physical obstacles. Here is the WHO definition of barriers:

"Factors in a person's environment that, through their absence or presence, limit functioning and create disability. These include aspects such as:

- a physical environment that is not accessible,

- lack of relevant assistive technology (assistive, adaptive, and rehabilitative devices),

- negative attitudes of people towards disability,

- services, systems and policies that are either nonexistent or that hinder the involvement of all people with a health condition in all areas of life."

Often there are multiple barriers that can make it extremely difficult or even impossible for people with disabilities to function. Here are the seven most common barriers. Often, more than one barrier occurs at a time.

- Attitudinal

- Communication

- Physical

About This Chapter: This chapter includes text excerpted from "Disability And Health: Disability Inclusion," National Center on Birth Defects and Developmental Disabilities (NCBDDD), Centers for Disease Control and Prevention (CDC), March 17, 2016.

- Policy

- Programmatic

- Social

- Transportation

Attitudinal Barriers

Attitudinal barriers are the most basic and contribute to other barriers. For example, some people may not be aware that difficulties in getting to or into a place can limit a person with a disability from participating in everyday life and common daily activities. Examples of attitudinal barriers include:

- **Stereotyping:** People sometimes stereotype those with disabilities, assuming their quality of life is poor or that they are unhealthy because of their impairments.

- **Stigma, prejudice, and discrimination:** Within society, these attitudes may come from people's ideas related to disability—people may see disability as a personal tragedy, as something that needs to be cured or prevented, as a punishment for wrongdoing, or as an indication of the lack of ability to behave as expected in society.

Today, society's understanding of disability is improving as we recognize "disability" as what occurs when a person's functional needs are not addressed in his or her physical and social environment. By not considering disability a personal deficit or shortcoming, and instead thinking of it as a social responsibility in which all people can be supported to live independent and full lives, it becomes easier to recognize and address challenges that all people—including those with disabilities—experience.

Communication Barriers

Communication barriers are experienced by people who have disabilities that affect hearing, speaking, reading, writing, and or understanding, and who use different ways to communicate than people who do not have these disabilities. Examples of communication barriers include:

- Written health promotion messages with barriers that prevent people with vision impairments from receiving the message. These include

- use of small print or no large-print versions of material, and

- no Braille or versions for people who use screen readers.

- Auditory health messages may be inaccessible to people with hearing impairments, including

- videos that do not include captioning, and

- oral communications without accompanying manual interpretation (such as, American Sign Language).

- The use of technical language, long sentences, and words with many syllables may be significant barriers to understanding for people with cognitive impairments.

Physical Barriers

Physical barriers are structural obstacles in natural or manmade environments that prevent or block mobility (moving around in the environment) or access. Examples of physical barriers include:

- Steps and curbs that block a person with mobility impairment from entering a building or using a sidewalk;

- Mammography equipment that requires a woman with mobility impairment to stand; and

- Absence of a weight scale that accommodates wheelchairs or others who have difficulty stepping up.

Policy Barriers

Policy barriers are frequently related to a lack of awareness or enforcement of existing laws and regulations that require programs and activities be accessible to people with disabilities. Examples of policy barriers include:

- Denying qualified individuals with disabilities the opportunity to participate in or benefit from federally funded programs, services, or other benefits;

- Denying individuals with disabilities access to programs, services, benefits, or opportunities to participate as a result of physical barriers; and

- Denying reasonable accommodations to qualified individuals with disabilities, so they can perform the essential functions of the job for which they have applied or have been hired to perform.

Programmatic Barriers

Programmatic barriers limit the effective delivery of a public health or healthcare program for people with different types of impairments. Examples of programmatic barriers include:

- Inconvenient scheduling;

- Lack of accessible equipment (such as mammography screening equipment);

- Insufficient time set aside for medical examination and procedures;

- Little or no communication with patients or participants; and

- Provider's attitudes, knowledge, and understanding of people with disabilities.

Social Barriers

Social barriers are related to the conditions in which people are born, grow, live, learn, work and age—or social determinants of health—that can contribute to decreased functioning among people with disabilities. Here are examples of social barriers:

- People with disabilities are far less likely to be employed. The unemployment rate in 2012 for people with disabilities was more than 1 in 10 (13.9%) compared to less than 1 in 10 (6.0%) for those without disabilities.

- Adults age 25 years and older with disabilities are less likely to have completed high school compared to their peers without disabilities (23.5% compared to 11.1%).

- People with disabilities are more likely to live in poverty compared to people without disabilities (21.6% compared to 12.8%).

- Children with disabilities are almost four times more likely to experience violence than children without disabilities.

Transportation Barriers

Transportation barriers are due to a lack of adequate transportation that interferes with a person's ability to be independent and to function in society. Examples of transportation barriers include:

- Lack of access to accessible or convenient transportation for people who are not able to drive because of vision or cognitive impairments, and

- Public transportation may be unavailable or at inconvenient distances or locations.

Inclusion Strategies

Inclusion of people with disabilities into everyday activities involves practices and policies designed to identify and remove barriers such as physical, communication, and attitudinal, that hamper individuals' ability to have full participation in society, the same as people without disabilities. Inclusion involves:

- getting fair treatment from others (nondiscrimination);

- making products, communications, and the physical environment more usable by as many people as possible (universal design);

- modifying items, procedures, or systems to enable a person with a disability to use them to the maximum extent possible (reasonable accommodations); and

- eliminating the belief that people with disabilities are unhealthy or less capable of doing things (stigma, stereotypes).

National Policy And Legislation

Three federal laws protect the rights of people with disabilities and ensure their inclusion in many aspects of society:

- Section 504 of the Rehabilitation Act of 1973

- The Americans with Disabilities Act (ADA) of 1990, which was followed by the ADA Amendments Act of 2008 in an attempt to restore the original intent of the legislation

- The Patient Protection and Affordable Care Act in 2010

Section 504 of the Rehabilitation Act

Section 504 of the Rehabilitation Act of 1973 is a federal law that protects individuals from discrimination based on disability. The nondiscrimination requirements of the law apply to employers and organizations that receive financial assistance from federal departments or agencies. Section 504 forbids organizations and employers from denying individuals with disabilities an equal opportunity to receive program benefits and services. It defines the rights of individuals with disabilities to participate in, and have access to, program benefits and services.

Americans with Disabilities Act

The Americans with Disabilities Act (ADA) of 1990, as amended, protects the civil rights of people with disabilities, and has helped remove or reduce many barriers for people with disabilities. The legislation required the elimination of discrimination against people with disabilities. The ADA has expanded opportunities for people with disabilities by reducing barriers, changing perceptions, and increasing participation in community life.

ADA guarantees equal opportunity for individuals with disabilities in several areas:

- employment
- public accommodations such as restaurants, hotels, theaters, doctors' offices, pharmacies, retail stores, museums, libraries, parks, private schools, and day care centers
- transportation
- state and local government services
- telecommunications such as telephones, televisions, and computers

People with Disabilities and the Patient Protection and Affordable Care Act

On March 23, 2010, President Obama signed into law the Patient Protection and Affordable Care Act, commonly referred as ACA.

For people with disabilities, the ACA:

- provides more healthcare choices and enhanced protection for Americans with disabilities;
- provides new healthcare options for long-term support and services;
- improves the Medicaid home- and community-based services option;
- provides access to high-quality and affordable healthcare for many people with disabilities;
- mandates accessible preventive screening equipment; and
- designates disability status as a demographic category and mandates data collection to assess health disparities.

Reasonable Accommodations

Accommodations are alterations that have been made to items, procedures, or systems that enable a person with a disability to use them to the maximum extent possible. An accommodation can also be a modification to an existing environment or process to increase the participation by an individual with an impairment or activity limitation. Braille, large print, or audio books are examples of accommodations for people who are blind or who have visual limitations otherwise. For people who are deaf or who have difficulty hearing, accommodations may take the form of having an American Sign Language interpreter available during meetings or presentations, or exchanging written messages. Communication accommodations do not have to be elaborated, but they must be able to convey information effectively.

Assistive Technology

Assistive technologies (ATs) are devices or equipment that can be used to help a person with a disability fully engage in life activities. ATs can help enhance functional independence and make daily living tasks easier through the use of aids that help a person travel, communicate with others, learn, work, and participate in social and recreational activities. An example of an assistive technology can be anything from a low-tech device, such as a magnifying glass, to a high-tech device, such as a computer that talks and helps someone communicate. Other examples are wheelchairs, walkers, and scooters, which are mobility aids that can be used by persons with physical disabilities. Smartphones have greatly expanded the availability of assistive technology for people with vision or hearing difficulties, or who have problems with effectively communicating their thoughts because of mental or physical limitations.

Chapter 48

Social Skills, Friends, And Dating

Not all of the effects of learning disabilities (LD) are related to academic success. In addition to school-related issues, teens with LD often experience difficulties with making friends and forming romantic relationships. Although the social skills involved in these personal interactions come naturally to many people, you may need help or training to develop these skills if you have learning or attention issues. This sort of training can provide important benefits in the classroom and contribute to successful relationships later in life.

Some learning and attention issues can have a direct impact on your social skills and lead to social isolation or rejection. If you struggle with visual or auditory perception, for instance, you may not notice or understand facial expressions, vocal inflection, or other social "cues" as easily as your peers. As a result, you may have trouble gauging and responding to the moods of people you interact with. If you have spatial awareness issues, you may struggle with the concept of personal space. You may stand closer to other people than they are comfortable with while talking to them. Some teens with attention issues may behave impulsively or disruptively without thinking through all the potential consequences of their actions. Others may have trouble setting realistic goals, being well-organized, and staying on task. These issues can create frustration for their classmates and negatively affect social relationships.

Building Social Skills

Fortunately, parents and teachers can help teens with LD learn strategies to deal with social situations. Special social skills training is also available through school- or community-based counseling services. By working to improve your social skills, you will be able to interact more

---

"Social Skills, Friends, And Dating," © 2017 Omnigraphics. Reviewed January 2017.

positively with your peers, which may also help improve your academic performance. Some of the techniques and strategies for teaching social skills include the following:

- **Role-playing**

  Role-playing enables you to learn about and practice using social conventions in a safe environment. Taking turns with an adult, you can think up situations that require good social skills and model appropriate responses. This technique can also be useful in helping you recognize facial expressions and interpret vocal tone. The adult can model certain moods or expressions and have you guess what they are. Another way to observe nonverbal behavior is by watching television with the sound muted and discussing what each character is trying to convey with their body language.

- **Body awareness**

  Teens with LD sometimes struggle with a lack of awareness of their body position. One strategy for addressing this issue is to perform everyday physical activities such as sitting down, standing up, climbing stairs, or eating while a parent records you with a video camera. Watching yourself on video can help you increase awareness of your physical positioning and reduce movements that may appear socially awkward.

- **Receiving information**

  Teens with LD often need to receive information in specific ways in order to remember or process it effectively. Asking for help in receiving information is an important social skill that should be developed in school. You can work with your teachers to learn polite methods of requesting information or accommodations. Instead of saying "I don't get it," for instance, the teacher might encourage you to say, "Could you please explain the directions to me again so I can be sure I understand?"

- **Organizational skills**

  Disorganization can make life more complicated for anyone. For teens with LD, however, it can lead to visual distraction, time-consuming searches, and frustrating delays. Learning to organize things is a valuable skill that can lead to improvements in many other areas. You can work with your parents and teachers to develop better organizational skills and strategies. For example, you might devise a system for putting everything you need for school in a specific place the night before to save time in the morning.

- **Conversation skills**

  It can be difficult for some teens with LD to understand the hidden rules of conversation. Without coping strategies, they may tend to dominate conversations or avoid participating completely. Social skills training can help you develop strategies for improving your conversational skills, such as making eye contact, nodding to show that you are listening, or looking puzzled if you need someone to explain something further. It may also be helpful to memorize a basic response to common questions, like "what do you do?" to make small talk easier.

Making Friends

The academic and social challenges facing teens with LD can make it difficult to form friendships. The skills required in making and keeping friends—such as talking, listening, sharing, and understanding—may not always come naturally to you. You may feel as if you don't fit in with your classmates, and you may wish that you were included in more group activities. Difficulty in making friends can impact your confidence and self-esteem and prevent you from getting involved in new things. In addition, research has shown that teens without close friends are more likely to drop out of school, abuse substances, and get in trouble with the law.

Fortunately, talking about your feelings with your parents can help you feel better about yourself. The strategies listed above can help you strengthen your social and communication skills, which can give you more confidence in connecting with other teens. It may also be helpful to ask your teachers to observe your interactions with classmates and provide feedback about your strengths and weaknesses. You can analyze various social interactions to determine what went well and identify areas to work on for next time. Finally, it is important to note that many friendships among teens are built upon shared interests in music, sports, computers, or other activities. You may be more likely to form lasting friendships by joining teams, clubs, or groups made up of people who share your interests.

Did You Know...
Studies have shown that 70 percent of students with LD report having "major difficulty" relating to their peers, compared to only 15 percent of nondisabled students.

Dating

For teens with LD who have trouble with ordinary social interactions, dating can be very challenging. The social cues involved in romantic relationships are even more confusing than those involved in platonic friendship. To develop the skills needed to have successful relationships, experts offering the following suggestions:

- **Find good role models**

   Happy couples can shed light on the secrets to forming solid, lasting relationships. Identify positive relationship role models among your family or friends and watch how they speak to and treat each other.

- **Observe dating interactions**

   There are many other examples of romantic social interaction—both positive and negative—on television, in the movies, at the mall, or in the hallways at school. You can observe these interactions for instructive lessons about human behavior, such as making eye contact, appropriate touching, and flirting.

- **Take failure in stride**

   The difficult truth is that most teenage romantic relationships are temporary. As a result, it can be helpful to view dating experiences as opportunities for self-reflection, learning, and improvement. Think about the positive and negative aspects of the interaction and use that information on your next date.

References

1. Brown, Dale S. "Finding Friends and Persuading People: Teaching the Skills of Social Interaction," LD Online, September-October 1987.

2. Hayes, Marnell L. "Social Skills: The Bottom Line for Adult LD Success," LD Online, 2015.

3. "How Learning and Attention Issues Can Cause Trouble with Making Friends," Understood, 2016.

4. Lavoie, Rick. "Helping the Socially Isolated Child Make Friends," LD Online, 2015.

5. Rosen, Peg. "At a Glance: Dating Hurdles for Teens with Learning and Attention Issues," Understood, 2016.

6. Sacks, Melinda. "The Challenges of Romance for Teens with LD," GreatSchools, October 14, 2016.

7. "Social Skills and Learning Disabilities," Learning Disabilities Association of America, 2017.

Chapter 49

Stopping Bullies

Bullying Among Children And Youth With Disabilities And Special Health Needs

Bullying is unwanted, aggressive behavior among school-aged children that involves a real or perceived power imbalance. The behavior is repeated, or has the potential to be repeated, over time. Both kids who are bullied and who bully others may have serious, lasting problems.

In order to be considered bullying, the behavior must be aggressive and include:

- **An imbalance of power:** Kids who bully use their power—such as physical strength, access to embarrassing information, or popularity—to control or harm others. Power imbalances can change over time and in different situations, even if they involve the same people.

- **Repetition:** Bullying behaviors happen more than once or have the potential to happen more than once.

> ## Types Of Bullying
> There are three types of bullying:
>
> - **Physical**
>   Physical bullying involves hurting a person's body or possessions. Physical bullying includes: hitting/kicking/pinching, spitting, tripping/pushing, taking or breaking someone's things, and making mean or rude hand gestures

About This Chapter: This chapter includes text excerpted from "Bullying Among Children And Youth With Disabilities And Special Health Needs," StopBullying.gov, U.S. Department of Health and Human Services (HHS), 2012. Reviewed December 2016.

- **Verbal**

  Verbal bullying is saying or writing mean things. Verbal bullying includes: teasing, name-calling, inappropriate sexual comments, taunting, and threatening to cause harm.

- **Social**

  Social bullying, sometimes referred to as relational bullying, involves hurting someone's reputation or relationships. Social bullying includes: leaving someone out on purpose, telling other children not to be friends with someone, spreading rumors about someone, or embarrassing someone in public.

Verbal and social bullying also can come in the form of electronic aggression (e.g., cyberbullying using the Internet or cell phones). It can include threatening, embarrassing, or insulting emails, texts.

What Is Known About Bullying Among Children With Disabilities And Special Needs?

Children with disabilities—such as physical, developmental, intellectual, emotional, and sensory disabilities—are at an increased risk of being bullied. Any number of factors—physical vulnerability, social skill challenges, or intolerant environments—may increase the risk. Research suggests that some children with disabilities may bully others as well.

Kids with special health needs, such as epilepsy or food allergies, also may be at higher risk of being bullied. Bullying can include making fun of kids because of their allergies or exposing them to the things they are allergic to. In these cases, bullying is not just serious, it can mean life or death.

Through a small but growing amount of research, we have learned that:

- Although little research has been conducted on the relation between learning disabilities (LD) and bullying, available information indicates that children with LD are at greater risk of being bullied. At least one study also has found that children with LD may also be more likely than other children to bullying their peers.

- Children with attention deficit or hyperactivity disorder (ADHD) are more likely than other children to be bullied. They also are somewhat more likely than others to bully their peers.

- Children with autism spectrum disorder (ASD) are at increased risk of being bullied and ostracized by peers. In a study of 8–17-year-olds, researchers found that children with ASD had bully victimization scores that were more than three times as high as students in a control group with no special needs.

- Children with epilepsy are more likely to be bullied by peers, as are children with medical conditions that affect their appearance (e.g., cerebral palsy, muscular dystrophy, and spina bifida). Frequently, these children report being called names related to their disability.

- Children with hemiplegia (paralysis of one side of their body) are more likely than other children their age to be victimized by peers, to be rated as less popular than their peers, and to have fewer friends than other children.

- Children who stutter may be more likely than their peers to be bullied. In one study, 83 percent of adults who had problems with stammering as children said that they had been teased or bullied; 71 percent of those who had been bullied said it happened at least once a week.

How Does Bullying Affect Children?

Kids who are bullied can experience negative physical, school, and mental health issues. Kids who are bullied are more likely to experience:

- Depression and anxiety, increased feelings of sadness and loneliness, changes in sleep and eating patterns, and loss of interest in activities they used to enjoy. These issues may persist into adulthood.

Other Effects of Bullying

Children and youth who are bullied are more likely than other children to:

- Have low self-esteem;
- Experience headaches, stomachaches, tiredness, and poor eating;
- Think about suicide or plan for suicide.

Some children with disabilities have low self-esteem or feel depressed, lonely or anxious because of their disability, and bullying may make this even worse. Bullying can cause serious, lasting problems not only for children who are bullied but also for children who bully and those who witness bullying.

(Source: "Safety and Children with Disabilities: Bullying," National Center on Birth Defects and Developmental Disabilities (NCBDDD), Centers for Disease Control and Prevention (CDC).)

- Health complaints

- Decreased academic achievement—GPA and standardized test scores—and school participation. They are more likely to miss, skip, or drop out of school.

Is Bullying Of Kids With Disabilities Covered By Federal Law?

Yes. Bullying behavior may cross the line to become **"disability harassment,"** which is prohibited under Section 504 of the Rehabilitation Act of 1973 and Title II of the Americans with Disabilities Act of 1990 (ADA). According to the U.S. Department of Education (ED), disability harassment is "intimidation or abusive behavior toward a student based on disability that creates a hostile environment by interfering with or denying a student's participation in or receipt of benefits, services, or opportunities in the institution's program" (ED, 2000). This behavior can take different forms including verbal harassment, physical threats, or threatening written statements. When a school finds out that harassment may have occurred, staff must investigate the incident(s) promptly and respond appropriately.

Disability harassment can occur in any location that is connected with school: in classrooms, in the cafeteria, in hallways, on the playground or athletic fields, or on a school bus. It also can occur during school-sponsored events.

What Can I Do If I Think My Child Is Being Bullied Or Is The Victim Of Disability Harassment?

- Be supportive of your child and encourage him or her to describe who was involved and how and where the bullying or harassment happened. Be sure to tell your child that it is not his or her fault and that nobody deserves to be bullied or harassed. Do not encourage your child to fight back. This may make the problem much worse.

- Usually children are able to identify when they are being bullied by their peers. Sometimes, however, children with disabilities do not realize they are being targeted. (They may, for example, believe that they have a new friend, when in fact, this "friend" is making fun of them.) Ask your child specific questions about his or her friendships and be alert to possible signs of bullying—even if your child doesn't label the behaviors as bullying.

- Talk with your child's teacher immediately to see whether he or she can help to resolve the problem quickly.

- If the bullying or harassment is severe, or if the teacher doesn't fix the problem quickly, contact the principal and put your concerns in writing. Explain what happened in detail and ask for a prompt response. Keep a written record of all conversations and communications with the school.

- Ask the school district to convene a meeting of the Individualized Education Program (IEP) team or the Section 504 team, a group convened to ensure that the school district is meeting the needs of its students with disabilities. This meeting will allow you to explain what has been happening and will let the team review your child's IEP or 504 plan and make sure that the school is taking steps to stop the harassment. If your child needs counseling or other supportive services because of the harassment, discuss this with the team.

- As the ED recognizes, "creating a supportive school climate is the most important step in preventing harassment." Work with the school to help establish a system-wide bullying prevention program that includes support systems for bullied children.

- Sometimes children and youth who are bullied also bully others. Explore whether your child may also be bullying other younger, weaker students at school. If so, his or her IEP may need to be modified to include help to change the aggressive behavior.

- Be persistent. Talk regularly with your child and with school staff to see whether the behavior has stopped.

Chapter 50
Siblings With Learning Disabilities

In any family, each sibling is unique, important, and special. So are the relationships they have with each other. Brothers and sisters influence each other and play important roles in each other's lives. Indeed, sibling relationships make up a child's first social network and are the basis for his or her interactions with people outside the family.

Brothers and sisters are playmates first; as they mature, they take on new roles with each other. Over the years, they may be many things to each other—teacher, friend, companion, follower, protector, enemy, competitor, confidant, role model. This relationship can be powerfully affected by a sibling's disability or chronic illness.

What do the sibs have to say about their experience of having a brother or sister with a disability? Read on, because they have a lot to say.

Brothers And Sisters, In Their Own Words

We know from the experiences of families and the findings of research that having a child with a disability powerfully affects everyone in the family. This includes that child's brothers and sisters. Many authors and researchers have written with eloquence about how the presence of a disability affects each sibling individually, as well as the relationships between siblings.

It's different for everyone. The impact of disability in the family varies considerably from person to person. Yet there are common threads that run through siblings' stories. For many, the experience is a positive, enriching one that teaches them to accept other people as they are. Some become deeply involved in helping parents care for the child with a disability. It is not

About This Chapter: This chapter includes text excerpted from "Sibling Issues," Center for Parent Information and Resources (CPIR), May 2014.

uncommon for siblings to become ardent protectors and supporters of their brother or sister with special needs or to experience feelings of great joy in watching him or her achieve even the smallest gain in learning or development.

Megan, age 17, says of her life with her brother who has Down syndrome:

Every day Andy teaches me to never give up. He knows he is different, but he doesn't focus on that. He doesn't give up, and every time I see him having a hard time, I make myself work that much harder…I don't know what I would do without Andy. He changed my life…If I had not grown up with him, I would have less understanding, patience, and compassion for people. He shows us that anyone can do anything.

In contrast, many siblings experience feelings of bitterness and resentment towards their parents or the brother or sister with a disability. They may feel jealous, neglected, or rejected as they watch most of their parents' energy, attention, money, and psychological support flow to the child with special needs. As Angela, age 8, puts it, *"[T]here are times when I sit down and think, 'It's not fair!'"*

And many, many siblings swing back and forth between positive and negative emotions. Helen, age 10, whose sister has severe intellectual disabilities and seizures, begins by saying that she's glad to have a sister with special needs.

- *"It has opened my eyes to a world of people I never would have known about."*

- But Helen also says, *"Sometimes I wish I had special needs. I think that a lot when Martha gets ooohed and aahed over and nobody even thinks about me."*

- Then in the next breath, Helen says, *"Another thing is that it really makes me mad when kids slap their chest with their hands and go, 'I'm a retard!' It made me so mad!"*

Age can make a difference. The reaction and adjustment of siblings to a brother or sister with a disability may also vary depending upon their ages and developmental levels. The younger the nondisabled sibling is, the more difficult it may be for him or her to understand the situation and to interpret events realistically. Younger children may be confused about the nature of the disability, including what caused it. They may feel that they themselves are to blame or may worry about "catching" the disability.

As siblings mature, their understanding of the disability matures as well, but new concerns may emerge. They may worry about the future of their brother or sister, about how their peers will react to their sibling, or about whether or not they themselves can pass the disability along to their own children.

Talking with your children about disability. Clearly, it is important for you to take time to talk openly about your child's disability with your other children, explaining it as best you can in terms that are appropriate to each child's developmental level.

If you're concerned about sibling issues, get in touch with resources that can help you open up the lines of communication and address the needs of your nondisabled children. You may also find there is a support group available to your children, which can provide an "excellent outlet" for siblings to share their feelings with others in a similar situation. The Internet also offers amazing possibilities for connection sharing.

Chapter 51

Becoming A Successful Adult

Transitioning From College To Work

Transitioning from college to work is a process. Students must begin this process early and be able to transfer knowledge of their learning disability (LD) into the world of employment.

Students should consider the following:

- What do I think the impact of the LD will be on my job performance?

- How or when should I disclose my LD?

- Do I know the typical accommodations made in the workforce?

- What kinds of social demands and interactions will I have?

Students must recognize the disability's impact on career choices. Knowledge of the disability and how it affects work are critical to getting and keeping a job individuals like and do well in. In addition to clearly understanding the disability, students need to identify goals. They must analyze training and career goals in relation to their disability. What kind of tasks will the job include? What kind of interaction between job tasks and the disability will need to be determined? When answering these questions, the student should assess the work environment, the type and amount of co-worker or peer interaction, specific tasks or essential functions that must be performed, and how performance is evaluated.

About This Chapter: Text in this chapter is excerpted from "Transitioning From College To Work," © 2016 Learning Disabilities Association of America (LDA). Reprinted with permission.

The Laws That Govern Employment

Students should become familiar with laws that identify their rights to equal access and non-discrimination. They should understand the aspects of the Americans with Disabilities Act Amendments Act (ADAAA) of 2008 and the Rehabilitation Act of 1973, Section 504, which assure equal access and non-discrimination. It is not enough to only know their legal rights. Students must recognize how equal access applies to them individually, within a particular education, employment or community setting, and in relation to the disability. They need to ask themselves the following questions:

- Is it necessary for me to disclose my disability in order to perform more efficiently?

- To whom do I disclose?

- How do I disclose?

- When do I disclose?

- How do I negotiate accommodations? And with whom?

Being able to describe the potential effect of the disability in relation to the work environment is central to successful employment. Individuals should know what accommodations might be needed (if any) in order to perform the required tasks or essential functions of the job.

Steps To Successful Employment

1. **Develop a history of work experience.** Look for opportunities to gain work experience. Some examples include:

   - campus leadership opportunities (e.g., student government, mentoring programs, organization involvement, etc.)

   - work-study positions on campus

   - internships

   - off-campus jobs (some may be listed in the college career center)

   - summer jobs

   - service learning opportunities

   - volunteer positions with community-based organizations and/or religious affiliations

   - job opportunities found through family and friends

2. **Understand the job culture.** Every company or organization has its own unique culture. The job culture consists of company rules, values, and beliefs, which are widely held but often unspoken.

   - Observe co-workers, not only how they work, but also how they communicate and interact.

   - Know what is expected of employees.

3. **Determine effective job accommodations.** Match job tasks or essential functions with strengths and weaknesses to identify potential accommodations that will improve job performance. Accommodations that may be used in the workplace include:

   - audio recorders (smart phone, smart pens, tablets, or other recording devices)

   - audio materials (for review when needed)

   - speech-to-text software or app

   - text-to-speech software or app

   - printed instructions

   - demonstration of tasks/assignments (record video with smartphone or tablet for multiple playbacks as needed)

   - diagrams to explain the process of an assigned task

   - separate or quiet workspace

   - computer software (e.g., word prediction, grammar-check, templates, etc.)

   - computer access with dual monitors

   - color-coding of files, work assignments, etc.

   - understanding how to use the software on the company's computer.

4. **Identify and use a support system.** Family, friends, and co-workers are vital to successful employment. A support system can be a valuable asset through the entire transition process from college to work.

5. **Devise an individual employment approach.** Individuals eligible for Vocational Rehabilitation Services (in some states also called Rehabilitation Services Administration, or RSA) can work with counselors to design an individualized plan

addressing employment, assessments, and services related to employment. This may also include employment training.

6. **Develop job skills.** Many workplaces will offer options for learning how to do the job. Some options to explore include:

   - coaching/mentoring

   - internships

7. **Seek assistance. Here are a few of the many resources that are available:**

   - Rehabilitation Services Administration, rsa.ed.gov

   - Equal Employment Opportunity Commission Helpline, www.eeoc.gov, 800-669-4000

   - HEATH Resource Center, www.heath.gwu.edu

   - Job Accommodation Network (JAN), askjan.org

   - National Rehabilitation Information Center, www.naric.com, 800-346-2742

   - Peterson's Internships, www.petersons.com

Chapter 52
Learning Disabilities On The Job

Youth With Learning Disabilities: The Challenges

Youth with learning disabilities (LD) face multiple challenges that complicate their training and learning trajectories. This following provides an overview of how learning disabilities impact employment and literacy development for youth.

Characteristics

Learning disabilities are a group of disorders that can impact many areas of learning, including reading, reading comprehension, writing, spelling, math, listening, oral expression, information processing and organization, with reading difficulties being the most common. Youth with LD demonstrate different types and degrees of difficulties and strengths. LDs are lifelong; they are not outgrown and often impact individuals in the workplace. It is important to note that many youth with LD lack a clear understanding of their disability and its potential impact on their ability to perform a job. As a result, many make poor career choices.

Employment Challenges

Being an employee is just one valued adult role, but it is a significant indicator of adult success and autonomy in the United States. Working is how people contribute to their

About This Chapter: Text under the heading "Youth With Learning Disabilities: The Challenges" is excerpted from "Literacy, Employment And Youth With Learning Disabilities: Aligning Workforce Development Policies And Programs," National Institute for Literacy (NIFL), U.S. Department of Education (ED), September 2010. Reviewed December 2016; Text under the heading "Disclosure And The Workplace: Why, When, What, And How" is excerpted from "Youth, Disclosure, And The Workplace Why, When, What, And How," Office of Disability Employment Policy (ODEP), U.S. Department of Labor (DOL), June 6, 2007. Reviewed December 2016; Text under the heading "Requesting Reasonable Accommodations At Work" is excerpted from "Disability: Reasonable Accommodation Process," Job Corps, U.S. Department of Labor (DOL), August 24, 2014.

communities and to the economy. The National Longitudinal Transition Study 2 (NLTS-2) (2003) findings indicate between 57 and 69 percent of youth with LD have the goal to attain competitive employment in their Individualized Education Program (IEP), and 43 percent would like to attend a vocational training program. While they value and strive for employment success, youth with LD often experience difficulties and require interventions in the workplace.

> The NLTS-2 found that only 46 percent of youth with LD actually had regular paid employment within two years of leaving high school.

Studies suggest that youth with LD experience high rates of unemployment and underemployment, fewer work hours, lower wages and lower annual incomes as adults than their nondisabled peers. According to the National Center for Learning Disabilities (NCLD), there are five common reasons why youth with LD experience challenges at work:

1. **Efficiency:** Slow pace of work, difficulties with organization.

2. **Accuracy:** High error rate associated with reading tasks and/or written correspondence.

3. **Sequencing of tasks:** Problems following instructions or completing projects with multiple steps.

4. **Time management:** Trouble with planning, being on time or meeting deadlines.

5. **Social skills:** Problems with meeting new people, with professional interactions and with discussing the impact of LD on tasks to be completed.

These are some of the predominant issues that limit the success of workers with LD, many of whom also struggle with "soft" skills and self-determination or empowerment skills. Below, we explore how these essential skills matter for youth with LD.

Soft Skills. While the "three R's" (reading, writing and arithmetic) are still fundamental to every employee's ability to do the job, employers view "soft" skills as even more important to work readiness. Youth frequently lack these skills, which include collaboration skills, critical thinking, problem-solving, and oral and written communication skills. According to a study, social skills are an important underpinning for success in any employment setting. These nonacademic limitations may have a greater adverse impact on achieving and maintaining employment than those associated with poor academic performance.

Self-Determination. The employment cycle characteristic of youth with LD is in part due to a lack of a focus on self-determination and empowerment by teachers, transition specialists, workplace programs and the youth themselves. Most youth and adults with LD do not receive needed accommodations on the job because they have chosen not to disclose their disability to their employer, reflecting a lack of self-awareness, self-determination, and self-advocacy. Self-disclosure to employers by working youth occurs only approximately 4 percent of the time. Many more youth do not accept that they have a learning disability or understand how it may impact their workplace performance, and therefore do not disclose their disability or request accommodations, leading to an unproductive working situation.

Literacy Challenges

Employment challenges for youth with LD are compounded by literacy needs. Many youth with LD have low literacy skills, especially in reading. The NLTS-2 found that reading achievement for youth with LD at the secondary school level is on average 3.4 years behind their enrolled grade level. Youth with LD, including those with undiagnosed LD, also often lack access to and training on explicit strategies for the use of assistive technology or adaptive equipment to access courses and reading materials to improve their literacy skills. Many such youth, therefore, enter workforce development programs and the workplace without the literacy skills, knowledge, supports and habits necessary for employment success. However, with appropriate supports and training, youth with LD can achieve and excel in the workplace.

To support literacy development, youth with LD who have extremely low basic literacy skills need multisensory, explicit, systematic, phonics-based instruction to enable them to learn to read and write proficiently. Small-group or one-on-one intense instruction may be required for youth who have not received LD-specific services through their school and who have extremely low literacy skills. This intensive and specific instruction is best delivered by trained literacy professionals.

Disclosure And The Workplace: Why, When, What, And How

Every job seeker with a disability is faced with the same decision: "Should I or shouldn't I disclose my disability?" This decision may be framed differently depending upon whether you have a visible disability or a non-visible disability. Ultimately, the decision of whether to disclose is entirely up to you.

Why Disclose In The Workplace?

When you leave school and enter the workforce, many aspects of your life change. Among the many differences, is the requirement to share information about your disability if you want your employer to provide you with reasonable accommodations (RA). In school if you had an IEP, as required under the Individuals with Disabilities Education Act (IDEA), information about your disability and the accommodations you needed followed you from grade to grade. When you enter the workforce, the IDEA no longer applies to you. Instead, the Americans with Disabilities Act (ADA) and the Rehabilitation Act protect you from disability-related discrimination and provide for meaningful access. The laws require that qualified applicants and employees with disabilities be provided with RA. Yet, in order to benefit from the ADA and the Rehabilitation Act, you must disclose your disability. An employer is only required to provide work-related accommodations if you disclose your disability to the appropriate individuals.

When To Disclose Your Disability

There is no one "right" time or place to disclose your disability. Select a confidential place in which to disclose, and allow enough time for the person to ask questions. Do not dwell on the limitations of your disability. You should weigh the pros and cons of disclosure at each point of the job search, recruitment, and hiring process and make the decision to discuss your disability when it is appropriate for you. Consider the following stages:

- In a letter of application or cover letter
- Before an interview
- At the interview
- In a third-party phone call or reference
- Before any drug testing for illegal drugs
- After you have a job offer
- During your course of employment or
- Never

How To Disclose Your Disability

Preparation is essential for disclosing your disability. Effective disclosure requires that you discuss your needs, and that you provide practical suggestions for reasonable job accommodations, if they are needed. One way to become comfortable with discussing your disability is to find someone you trust and practice the disclosure discussion with that person. The two of you can put together a disclosure script. It should contain relevant disability information and weave in your strengths. Always keep it positive!

What To Disclose About Your Disability

There is no required information to share about your disability. In fact, it will be different for everyone. For example, if you have an apparent disability it is often beneficial to address how you plan to accomplish tasks required by the job. This can affirm to the employer that you are suited for the position. Additionally, by demonstrating your own ease and comfort with the job requirements, you can relay to employers other traits that are desirable in an applicant. A person with a hidden disability, on the other hand, will first need to decide whether to disclose the disability, and subsequently determine what information to share about the disability. Generally, if you choose to disclose, it is most helpful to share the following:

- General information about your disability;

- Why you are disclosing your disability;

- How your disability affects your ability to perform key job tasks;

- Types of accommodations that have worked for you in the past; and

- Types of accommodations you anticipate needing in the workplace.

To Whom To Disclose Your Disability

Disclose your disability on a "need-to-know" basis. Provide further details about your disability as it applies to your work-related accommodations to the individual who has the authority to facilitate your accommodation request. Consider disclosing to the supervisor responsible for the hiring, promoting, and/or firing of employees. This person needs to be informed of your disability-related needs to provide the necessary supports and judge your job performance fairly.

Disclosure Protections And Responsibilities

As a person with a disability, you have disclosure protections as well as significant responsibilities to yourself and to your employers.

You are entitled to:

- Have information about your disability treated confidentially and respectfully;

- Seek information about hiring practices from any organization;

- Choose to disclose your disability at any time during the employment process;

- Receive RA for an interview;

- Be considered for a position based on your skill and merit; and

- Have respectful questioning about your disability for the purpose of determining whether you need accommodations and if so, what kind.

You have the responsibility to:

- Disclose your need for any work-related RA;

- Bring your skills and merits to the table; and

- Be truthful, self-determined, and proactive.

Requesting Reasonable Accommodations At Work

RAs are any changes to the environment or in the way things are customarily done, that give a person with a disability an opportunity to participate in the application process, job, program, or activity that is equal to the opportunity given to similarly situated people without disabilities. Although many people with disabilities can (and do) apply for and participate in

---

Who Can Request A Reasonable Accommodation?

An applicant for employment may request an RA, either orally or in writing, from any EPA employee authorized to interact with the applicant in the application process, the National Reasonable Accommodation Coordinator, or the Local Reasonable Accommodation Coordinator.

An employee, or an individual acting on behalf of the employee, may request an RA either orally or in writing, from his/her supervisor, another supervisor in his/her immediate chain of command, or the Reasonable Accommodation Coordinator in the office. When an RA request is made by a third party on behalf of an individual, the Agency official processing the request should confirm the individual's authority to represent the employee with a disability.

(Source: "Reasonable Accommodation," U.S. Environmental Protection Agency (EPA).)

---

a program without any RA, barriers do exist that keep other potential applicants or students with disabilities from applying or participating, and that could be overcome with some form of accommodation. RA may involve providing an appropriate service or product; modifying or adjusting a job, work/academic environment, policy, program, or procedure; or any other action that removes those barriers for the person with a disability.

Part Seven
Learning Disabilities And Your Legal Rights

Chapter 53

Laws That Protect People With Learning Disabilities

Introduction To The ADA

The Americans with Disabilities Act (ADA) was signed into law on July 26, 1990, by President George H.W. Bush. The ADA is one of America's most comprehensive pieces of civil rights legislation that prohibits discrimination and guarantees that people with disabilities have the same opportunities as everyone else to participate in the mainstream of American life—to enjoy employment opportunities, to purchase goods and services, and to participate in State and local government programs and services. Modeled after the Civil Rights Act of 1964, which prohibits discrimination on the basis of race, color, religion, sex, or national origin—and Section 504 of the Rehabilitation Act of 1973—the ADA is an "equal opportunity" law for people with disabilities.

To be protected by the ADA, one must have a disability, which is defined by the ADA as *a physical or mental impairment that substantially limits one or more major life activities, a person who has a history or record of such an impairment, or a person who is perceived by others as having such an impairment.* The ADA does not specifically name all of the impairments that are covered.

About This Chapter: Text under the heading "Introduction To The ADA" is excerpted from "Introduction To The ADA," U.S. Department of Justice (DOJ), May 17, 2013. Reviewed December 2016; Text beginning with the heading "Section 504 And The ADA" is excerpted from "Helping The Student With Diabetes Succeed: A Guide For School Personnel," The National Diabetes Education Program (NDEP), National Institute of Diabetes and Digestive and Kidney Diseases (NIDDK), November 2012. Reviewed December 2016.

Section 504 And The ADA*

Section 504 of the Rehabilitation Act of 1973 (Section 504) prohibits recipients of Federal financial assistance from discriminating against people on the basis of disability. Title II of the ADA prohibits discrimination on the basis of disability by public entities, regardless of whether the public entities receive Federal financial assistance. Public school districts that receive Federal financial assistance are covered by both Title II and Section 504, and the obligations of public schools to students with disabilities under each law are generally the same. For schools, these laws are enforced by the Office for Civil Rights (OCR) in the U.S. Department of Education (ED).

Section 504 outlines a process for schools to use in determining whether a student has a disability and in determining what services a student with a disability needs. This evaluation process must be tailored individually because each student is different and his or her needs will vary.

Under Section 504, students with disabilities must be given an equal opportunity to participate in academic, nonacademic, and extracurricular activities. The regulations also require school districts to identify all students with disabilities and to provide them with a free appropriate public education (FAPE). Under Section 504, FAPE is the provision of regular or special education and related aids and services designed to meet the individual educational needs of students with disabilities as adequately as the needs of students who do not have disabilities are met.

A student does not have to receive special education services, however, in order to receive related aids and services under Section 504. The most common practice is to include these related aids and services as well as any needed special education services in a written document, sometimes called a "Section 504 Plan."

Private schools that receive Federal financial assistance may not exclude an individual student with a disability if the school can, with minor adjustments, provide an appropriate education to that student. Private, nonreligious schools are covered by Title III of the ADA.

Both the Rehabilitation Act of 1973 and the Americans with Disabilities Act of 1990 (ADA) were amended by the ADA Amendments Act of 2008, P.L. 110–325.

Individuals with Disabilities Education Act (IDEA)

IDEA provides Federal funds to assist State educational agencies and, through them, local educational agencies in making special education and related services available to eligible children with disabilities. IDEA is administered by the Office of Special Education Programs (OSEP) in the Office of Special Education and Rehabilitative Services (OSERS) in the ED.

A child with a disability must meet the criteria of one or more of 13 disability categories and need special education and related services. IDEA requires school districts to find and identify children with disabilities and to provide them a FAPE. Under IDEA, FAPE means special education and related services that meet State standards and are provided in conformity with an Individualized Education Program (IEP). The IDEA regulations specify how school personnel and the parents/guardian, working together, develop and implement an IEP.

Each child's IEP must include the supplementary aids and services to be provided for or on behalf of the child and a statement of the program modifications or supports for school personnel that will be provided for the child to make progress and to be involved in the general education curriculum.

In general and consistent with the Family Educational Rights and Privacy Act (FERPA), IDEA's confidentiality provisions require prior written consent for disclosures of personally identifiable information contained in education records, unless a specific exception applies.

Chapter 54

Individuals with Disabilities Education Act (IDEA)

What Is The Individuals with Disabilities Education Act?[1]

The Individuals with Disabilities Education Act (IDEA) is the federal law dealing with the education of children with disabilities. Congress first passed IDEA in 1975, recognizing the need to provide a federal law to help ensure that local schools would serve the educational needs of students with disabilities. The law originally passed was titled the Education for All Handicapped Children Act. That first special education law has undergone several updates over the past 30 years. In 1990 the law got a new name—the Individuals with Disabilities Education Act (EHA), or IDEA. The most recent version of IDEA was passed by Congress in 2004. It can be referred to as either IDEA 2004 or IDEA.

In updating IDEA in 2004, Congress found that the education of students with disabilities has been impeded by "low expectations and an insufficient focus on applying replicable research on proven methods of teaching and learning…." Significant changes to IDEA as well as a close alignment to the No Child Left Behind Act (NCLB) are designed to provide students with disabilities access to high expectations and to the general education curriculum in the regular classroom, to the maximum extent possible, in order to "meet developmental goals and, to the extent possible, the challenging expectations that have been established for all children…."

IDEA serves 6.1 million school age children and almost 1 million children ages birth to 5.

About This Chapter: This chapter includes text excerpted from documents published by two sources. Text under headings marked 1 are excerpted from "NCLB and IDEA: What Parents Of Students With Disabilities Need To Know And Do," IDEAs That Work, U.S. Office of Special Education Programs (OSEP), August 2006. Reviewed January 2017; Text under heading marked 2 is © 2017 Omnigraphics. Reviewed January 2017.

> "The purposes of this title are to ensure that all children with disabilities have available to them a free appropriate public education that emphasizes special education and related services designed to meet their unique needs and prepare them for further education, employment and independent living...." *says Individuals with Disabilities Education Improvement Act of 2004.*

Six Principles Of Individuals with Disabilities Education Act[2]

The Individuals with Disabilities Education Act (IDEA) is a U.S. law enacted to ensure that children with disabilities are provided with the same "equality of opportunity, full participation, independent living, and economic self-sufficiency" as those without disabilities. In 1990 this legislation replaced the 1975 Education for All Handicapped Children Act (EHA), and since then it has been amended several times.

There are four distinct parts to IDEA. Part A describes the general provisions of the act and establishes the Office of Special Education Programs, which is responsible for administering the law. Part B creates educational guidelines for all school-age children with disabilities. Part C covers children from birth to age three. And Part D describes programs and activities created at the federal level to support children with disabilities.

IDEA sets forth six main principles, which have essentially been in place since 1975, and with which state and local school districts must comply if they are to receive federal funding:

Free Appropriate Public Education (FAPE)

IDEA requires that all children, regardless of severity or type of disability, receive an education without cost to their parents, other than normal costs assessed to all students, and that the educational services be appropriate to the student's "unique needs and prepare them for further education, employment, and independent living." To this end, an Individualized Education Program (IEP) must be developed for each student, specifying his or her needs and describing the educational services that will be provided to help the student progress in the general education curriculum.

Appropriate Evaluation

This principle is in place for two reasons: first, to ensure that the student is eligible according to the IDEA definition of a disability, and second, to determine his or her particular educational needs so that an appropriate IEP can be developed. The evaluation must include relevant information from a number of sources, including parents, teachers, classroom observation, and formal testing by experts. Schools are required to provide the evaluation free of charge, and if parents disagree with the conclusions, they have the right to request an independent evaluation, also without charge. They may also get an independent evaluation at their own expense at any time.

Individualized Education Program (IEP)

The IEP is a written, legal document developed by an IEP team made up of parents, educators, specialists, and the student, when appropriate. It must include an assessment of the student's current educational performance, measurable annual goals, short-term objectives, and an account of the student's participation in the general curriculum. It also describes the special educational services and support the student will receive and how they will help him or her meet specific goals and objectives. IDEA requires the IEP to be reviewed and revised at least annually by the IEP team, but it is a living document that may be reviewed as often as necessary throughout the year.

Least Restrictive Environment (LRE)

IDEA requires that students with disabilities be educated alongside those without disabilities as much as possible and that those with disabilities be moved to separate classrooms or buildings only when the severity of their condition would prevent them from receiving an appropriate education otherwise. Thus, the team and the school must make every effort to provide the necessary modifications, supplementary aid, special materials, and support needed for the student to succeed in the general educational environment. If this is not possible, plans must be made for the best possible LRE for the student outside of the regular classroom.

Parent And Student Participation In Decision Making

When IDEA was reauthorized in 2014, it was amended to make it clear that parents and, whenever possible, the student are full and equal participants in the education process. As a result, state agencies and local school boards are required to include parents of students with disabilities in any group or meeting that will make decisions about their child's IEP or LRE. They are also entitled to receive timely notice of relevant meetings, request that meetings be rescheduled so they can attend, approve or refuse additional evaluations of the student, and approve the release of any information about their child.

Procedural Safeguards

IDEA establishes a number of safeguards to protect the rights of children with disabilities and their parents and to ensure that they have access to all the information they need to participate in the educational process. For example, the school must provide parents with an annual written parental rights notice containing information about the special education process, procedural safeguards, and the rights of students and parents under the law. Parents also have the right to receive written notice prior to any evaluation or educational placement of their child, inspect and obtain copies of the student's records, and place an explanatory statement or correction in the record if they choose to do so. When parents disagree with any decisions related to their child, they have to right request mediation by an impartial third party. If the disagreement is not resolved, they can ask for a due-process hearing at the state level and, further, appeal the decision in state or federal court.

References

1. Heward, W.L. "Six Major Principles of IDEA," Education.com, July 19, 2013.

2. Lee, Andrew M.I., J.D. "How IDEA Protects You and Your Child," Understood.org, n.d.

3. Saleh, Matthew, J.D., M.S. "Your Child's Rights: 6 Principles of IDEA," Smart Kids with Learning Disabilities, n.d.

4. "Six Principles of IDEA: The Individuals With Disabilities Education Act, ASK Resource Center, 2013.

5. "6 Principles of IDEA," Parents Reaching Out, n.d.

What All States Must Do[1]

IDEA requires all states that accept IDEA funds to provide FAPE to all children with disabilities in the state. To achieve that goal, every state is required to:

- Establish a goal of providing full educational opportunity to all children with disabilities and a timetable for accomplishing that goal.

- Identify, locate, and evaluate all children with disabilities residing in the state who are in need of special education and related services.

- Ensure that all special education teachers are highly qualified.

- Evaluate every child suspected of having a disability in accordance with the requirements of IDEA.

- Annually develop an IEP for each child with a disability.

- Provide education services in the least restrictive environment—removing children from the regular education environment only when the nature or severity of their disability makes it necessary to do so.

- Provide all procedural safeguards required by IDEA to children with disabilities and their parents.

- Establish goals for the performance of children with disabilities that are the same as the state's definition of adequate yearly progress (AYP) and are consistent with any other goals and standards for children established by the state.

- Include all children with disabilities in all general state and districtwide assessment programs, including those assessments required by NCLB—students must be given appropriate accommodations and alternate assessments as indicated in their IEPs

The special education provided to children with disabilities must be specially designed instruction to meet the unique needs resulting from the child's disability and must enable the child to be involved and make progress in the general education curriculum.

IDEA: The Bottom Line[1]

Requirements of IDEA are designed to ensure that all schools, school districts, and states provide a FAPE to children with disabilities. IDEA focuses on the individual child—requiring the development of an IEP outlining the specially designed instruction necessary to allow the child to participate and progress in the same curriculum as all children.

However, nothing in IDEA holds schools accountable for the progress and performance of children with disabilities. While IDEA allows parents to challenge the adequacy of special education services, the law does not contain any measures of total school performance for IDEA-eligible students, as is required by NCLB.

> "State rules, regulations, and policies under this title shall support and facilitate local educational agency and school-level system improvement designed to enable children with disabilities to meet the challenging State student academic achievement standards." *says Individuals with Disabilities Education Improvement Act of 2004.*

Chapter 55

Protection For People With Learning Disabilities: Section 504 of the Rehabilitation Act

Section 504 of the Rehabilitation Act of 1973 protects the rights of persons with handicaps in programs and activities that receive Federal financial assistance. Section 504 protects the rights not only of individuals with visible disabilities but also those with disabilities that may not be apparent.

> Section 504 provides that: "No otherwise qualified individual with handicaps in the United States ... shall, solely by reason of her or his handicap, be excluded from the participation in, be denied the benefits of, or be subjected to discrimination under any program or activity receiving Federal financial assistance...."

The U.S. Department of Education (ED) enforces Section 504 in programs and activities that receive financial assistance from ED. Recipients of this assistance include public school districts, institutions of higher education, and other state and local education agencies.

Disabilities Covered Under Section 504

The ED Section 504 regulation defines an "individual with handicaps" as any person who

- has a physical or mental impairment which substantially limits one or more major life activities,

About This Chapter: This chapter includes text excerpted from "The Civil Rights Of Students With Hidden Disabilities Under Section 504 of the Rehabilitation Act of 1973," Office for Civil Rights (OCR), U.S. Department of Education (ED), October 15, 2015.

- has a record of such an impairment, or

- is regarded as having such an impairment.

The regulation further defines a physical or mental impairment as

- any physiological disorder or condition, cosmetic disfigurement, or anatomical loss affecting one or more of the following body systems: neurological; musculoskeletal; special sense organs; respiratory, including speech organs; cardiovascular; reproductive; digestive; genitourinary; hemic and lymphatic; skin; and endocrine; or

- any mental or psychological disorder, such as mental retardation, organic brain syndrome, emotional or mental illness, and specific learning disabilities. The definition does not set forth a list of specific diseases and conditions that constitute physical or mental impairments because of the difficulty of ensuring the comprehensiveness of any such list.

The key factor in determining whether a person is considered an "individual with handicaps" covered by Section 504 is whether the physical or mental impairment results in a substantial limitation of one or more major life activities. Major life activities, as defined in the regulation, include functions such as caring for one's self, performing manual tasks, walking, seeing, hearing, speaking, breathing, learning, and working.

The impairment must have a material effect on one's ability to perform a major life activity.

What Are Hidden Disabilities?

Hidden disabilities are physical or mental impairments that are not readily apparent to others. They include such conditions and diseases as specific learning disabilities, diabetes, epilepsy, and allergy. A disability such as a limp, paralysis, total blindness or deafness is usually obvious to others. But hidden disabilities such as low vision, poor hearing, heart disease, or chronic illness may not be obvious. A chronic illness involves a recurring and long-term disability such as diabetes, heart disease, kidney and liver disease, high blood pressure, or ulcers.

Approximately four million students with disabilities are enrolled in public elementary and secondary schools in the United States. Of these 43 percent are students classified as learning disabled, 8 percent as emotionally disturbed, and 1 percent as other health impaired. These hidden disabilities often cannot be readily known without the administration of appropriate diagnostic tests.

How Can The Needs Of Students With Hidden Disabilities Be Addressed?

The following examples illustrate how schools can address the needs of their students with hidden disabilities.

- A student with a long-term, debilitating medical problem such as cancer, kidney disease, or diabetes may be given special consideration to accommodate the student's needs. For example, a student with cancer may need a class schedule that allows for rest and recuperation following chemotherapy.

- A student with a learning disability that affects the ability to demonstrate knowledge on a standardized test or in certain testing situations may require modified test arrangements, such as oral testing or different testing formats.

- A student with a learning disability or impaired vision that affects the ability to take notes in class may need a notetaker or tape recorder.

- A student with a chronic medical problem such as kidney or liver disease may have difficulty in walking distances or climbing stairs. Under Section 504, this student may require special parking space, sufficient time between classes, or other considerations, to conserve the student's energy for academic pursuits.

- A student with diabetes, which adversely affects the body's ability to manufacture insulin, may need a class schedule that will accommodate the student's special needs.

- An emotionally or mentally ill student may need an adjusted class schedule to allow time for regular counseling or therapy.

- A student with epilepsy who has no control over seizures, and whose seizures are stimulated by stress or tension, may need accommodation for such stressful activities as lengthy academic testing or competitive endeavors in physical education.

- A student with arthritis may have persistent pain, tenderness or swelling in one or more joints. A student experiencing arthritic pain may require a modified physical education program.

These are just a few examples of how the needs of students with hidden disabilities may be addressed. If you are a student (or a parent or guardian of a student) with a hidden disability, or represent an institution seeking to address the needs of such students, you may wish to seek further information from Office For Civil Rights (OCR).

Chapter 56

Americans with Disabilities Act (ADA)

The Americans with Disabilities Act (ADA) outlaws discrimination and guarantees that people with disabilities have the same opportunities as everyone else to participate in all aspects of everyday life—to benefit from employment opportunities, to purchase goods and services and to participate in their state and local governments' programs and services. The ADA is one of several laws that protect the employment and other rights of people with disabilities.

The ADA is divided into the five sections or "titles" listed below. For the purposes of the ADA, a disability means a physical or mental impairment that substantially limits one or more major life activities; a person who has a history or record of that kind of impairment; or a person who is viewed by others as having such an impairment. The ADA does not specifically name all of the impairments or disabilities that it covers, but you'll see below under Title V that it does mention conditions that are not considered disabilities.

Below is a breakdown of some of what each of these titles of the ADA cover.

- **Employment:**

    Title I of the ADA protects the rights of employees and people looking for jobs. One of the key non-discrimination aspects of Title I is the legal requirement to provide reasonable accommodations for employees and job seekers with disabilities. Accommodations make it possible for a person with a disability to perform their job, but they must not create an "undue hardship" for the employer, in other words cause too much difficulty or expense to implement. What are some examples of reasonable accommodations that

About This Chapter: This chapter includes text excerpted from "Americans with Disabilities Act (ADA)," Disability. gov, U.S. Department of Labor (DOL), May 20, 2014.

may be needed during the hiring process? They can take many forms, including providing written materials in accessible formats, such as large print, Braille, or audiotape and providing readers or sign language interpreters.

An individual with a disability is a person who:

- has a physical or mental impairment that substantially limits one or more major life activities;
- has a record of such an impairment; or
- is regarded as having such an impairment.

A qualified employee or applicant with a disability is an individual who, with or without reasonable accommodation, can perform the essential functions of the job in question. Reasonable accommodation may include, but is not limited to:

- making existing facilities used by employees readily accessible to and usable by persons with disabilities.
- job restructuring, modifying work schedules, reassignment to a vacant position;
- acquiring or modifying equipment or devices, adjusting or modifying examinations, training materials, or policies, and providing qualified readers or interpreters.

(Source: "Facts About The Americans with Disabilities Act," U.S. Equal Employment Opportunity Commission (EEOC).)

This section of the law also makes it illegal for private employers, state and local governments, employment agencies and labor unions to discriminate against qualified individuals with disabilities in job application procedures, hiring, firing, promotions, wages and compensation and job training. Title I also prohibits employers from retaliating against someone who objects to employment practices that discriminate based on disability, or for filing a discrimination charge under the ADA. This section of the ADA is enforced by the U.S. Equal Employment Opportunity Commission (EEOC), and it applies to employers with 15 or more employees, including state and local governments.

Title I of the ADA is one of several laws that protect the employment rights of people with disabilities.

- **Public Services:**

  Title II of the ADA prohibits discrimination against qualified individuals with disabilities in all programs, activities, and services of public entities. The term "public entities" basically means any state or local government and any of its departments, agencies, offices or programs. The goal of Title II is really to make sure that people with disabilities have equal access to civic life. Individuals with disabilities must be allowed to have the same opportunity to participate in a public entity's programs and services the same as anyone else. This means having access to everything that a state or local government offers, including public housing, courts, all levels of public education, transportation, parks and recreation, emergency response and police.

> Unlike section 504 of the Rehabilitation Act of 1973, which only covers programs receiving federal financial assistance, Title II covers all the activities of state and local governments, whether or not they receive federal money. Title II also makes clear the requirements of Section 504 of the Rehabilitation Act as it relates to public transportation systems (city buses and subways) that receive federal financial assistance, as well as all public entities that provide public transportation.

States and local governments also have obligations under the ADA to make sure that websites, online job applications, e-learning courses and other technology are accessible for people with disabilities.

- **Public Accommodations:**

  Title III of the ADA prohibits public accommodations like hotels, golf courses, restaurants, parking, movie theaters, museums, daycare centers, doctor's offices and so on from discriminating against people with disabilities by having their establishments inaccessible to them. This section of the law sets the minimum standards for accessibility and design standards for alterations and new construction of facilities. It also requires these establishments to get rid of barriers in existing buildings when it can be done without much difficulty or expense. The U.S. Access Board develops accessibility guidelines and standards that apply to several other areas, including communications technologies, recreational facilities, transportation and access to healthcare and medical equipment used in doctors' offices and hospitals.

  Title III also directs businesses to make "reasonable modifications" when serving people with disabilities. They must take the necessary steps to communicate effectively with customers with vision, hearing and speech disabilities. For example, in the case of healthcare providers, they have a duty to provide appropriate auxiliary aids and services when needed in order to make sure that communication with people who are deaf or hard of hearing is as effective as communication with others. In addition, businesses and

309

nonprofit organizations that serve the public usually have to let people who use service animals bring their animal with them to public areas.

There are tax credits and deductions available to small businesses to help them remove barriers and make their places of business accessible to people with disabilities. Title III of the ADA is regulated and enforced by the U.S. Department of Justice (DOJ).

- **Telecommunications:**

  Title IV of the ADA requires telephone and Internet companies to provide a nation-wide system of telecommunications relay services that allow people with hearing and speech disabilities to communicate over the telephone. This title, which is regulated by the Federal Communications Commission, also requires closed captioning of federally funded public service announcements.

  There are several other laws that protect the rights of people with disabilities to access and use technology, including Section 255 of the Communications Act, Section 508 of the Rehabilitation Act, and, more recently, the 21st Century Communications and Video Accessibility Act. These services include emergency communications services, such as extreme weather alerts and warnings.

- **Miscellaneous Provisions:**

  Title V of the ADA:

  This last section of the ADA lists several requirements that relate to the ADA overall, including its relationship to other laws, prohibition against retaliation and coercion, illegal use of drugs, and attorney's fees. Title V also has a list of certain conditions that are not considered disabilities. For example, people who have sexual behavioral disorders, compulsive gambling, kleptomania, substance use disorders resulting from illegal use of drugs—these, among other conditions, are not considered disabilities to be protected under the ADA.

  The ADA Amendments Act of 2008:

  You may have heard people talk about the "new ADA." What they are actually refer-ring to is the ADA Amendments Act of 2008 (ADAAA), which overturns a series of Supreme Court decisions that interpreted the Americans with Disabilities Act of 1990 in a way that made it difficult to prove that an impairment is a disability. The ADAAA made important changes to the ADA's definition of "disability" that broadens the scope of coverage under both the ADA and Section 503 of the Rehabilitation Act. Whether a person had a disability (for example, being deaf) in order to sue became the focus of most disputes under the ADA. Congress never intended for it to be that way. The focus of the ADA was supposed to be on access and accommodation, not on whether the person really had a disability. So the ADAAA was passed in 2008 and overturned those Supreme Court cases that narrowed the definition of disability.

Filing a Complaint:

If you feel your rights have been violated, you can file an ADA complaint online or by calling the DOJ ADA Information Line at 800-514-0301 (TTY: 800-514-0383).

Title I of the ADA also covers:

- **Medical examinations and inquiries**

  Employers may not ask job applicants about the existence, nature, or severity of a disability. Applicants may be asked about their ability to perform specific job functions. A job offer may be conditioned on the results of a medical examination, but only if the examination is required for all entering employees in similar jobs. Medical examinations of employees must be job-related and consistent with the employer's business needs.

  Medical records are confidential. The basic rule is that with limited exceptions, employers must keep confidential any medical information they learn about an applicant or employee. Information can be confidential even if it contains no medical diagnosis or treatment course and even if it is not generated by a health care professional. For example, an employee's request for a reasonable accommodation would be considered medical information subject to the ADA's confidentiality requirements.

- **Drug and Alcohol Abuse**

  Employees and applicants currently engaging in the illegal use of drugs are not covered by the ADA when an employer acts on the basis of such use. Tests for illegal drugs are not subject to the ADA's restrictions on medical examinations. Employers may hold illegal drug users and alcoholics to the same performance standards as other employees.

It is also unlawful to retaliate against an individual for opposing employment practices that discriminate based on disability or for filing a discrimination charge, testifying, or participating in any way in an investigation, proceeding, or litigation under the ADA.

(Source: "Facts About The Americans with Disabilities Act," U.S. Equal Employment Opportunity Commission (EEOC).)

Learning Disabilities And The Law After High School: An Overview For Students

Do The Legal Rights Of Students With Learning Disabilities Continue After High School?

Legal rights may continue. It depends upon the facts in the individual case. Children with learning disabilities (LDs) who receive services under the Individuals with Disabilities Education Act (IDEA) or the Rehabilitation Act of 1973 in public elementary and secondary school may continue to have legal rights under federal laws in college programs and in employment. When students graduate from high school or reach age 21, their rights under the IDEA come to an end.

The rights that may continue are those under the Rehabilitation Act and the Americans with Disabilities Act of 1990 (ADA). To understand which rights continue, it is important to understand the three basic federal statutes that confer rights on people with disabilities.

The IDEA, initially enacted in 1975, provides for special education and related services for children with disabilities who need such education and services by reason of their disabilities. The IDEA provides for a Free Appropriate Public Education (FAPE) and for an Individualized Education Program (IEP).

The Rehabilitation Act, most notably Section 504, prohibits discrimination against children and adults with disabilities. The Rehabilitation Act applies to public and private elementary

About This Chapter: Text in this chapter is excerpted from "Learning Disabilities And The Law: After High School: An Overview For Students," © 2016 Learning Disabilities Association of America (LDA). Reprinted with permission.

and secondary schools and colleges that receive federal funding. It also applies to employers that receive federal funding.

The ADA prohibits discrimination against children and adults with disabilities and applies to all public and most private schools and colleges, to testing entities, and to licensing authorities, regardless of federal funding. Religiously controlled educational institutions are exempt from coverage. The ADA applies to private employers with 15 or more employees and to state and local governments.

> It may help to consider an example of how rights may continue over many years.
>
> Jeff has a reading disorder. For a long time he wanted to become a lawyer, and now he is in law school. He received special education and related services under the IDEA during public elementary school. He went to a small private religious high school and received accommodations under Section 504 of the Rehabilitation Act. He received extra test time on the SAT, during college, on the law school admission test (LSAT), and in law school. Under the ADA, he will be entitled to extra test time on the Bar Examination.

Do All People With Learning Disabilities Have Legal Rights Under The Rehabilitation Act And ADA?

No. Many have legal rights, but some do not. Under the Rehabilitation Act and ADA, a disability is an impairment that substantially limits a major life activity, such as learning. Children and adults with LDs, in many cases, have been found to have an impairment that substantially limits learning. That substantial limitation means that these individuals have a disability under the Rehabilitation Act and ADA and are protected under these laws.

Let's look at an example. Jim was diagnosed with a reading disorder and math disorder when he was six years old. He received special education under the IDEA for most of elementary school to assist with reading and math. By the time he entered high school, his reading comprehension and speed tested as average, but he continued to receive services under the IDEA for his math disorder through the end of high school. After graduation, Jim enrolled in art school. The art school required one math course as a requirement for graduation, but had a policy allowing course substitutions for the math requirement for students with disabilities that interfered with math. Jim disclosed his math disorder, requested a course substitution for math, and submitted good professional documentation of his disability and his need for accommodation.

What Rights Do I Have Under The Rehabilitation Act And ADA As A Person With A Disability?

Basically you have the right to be free from discrimination on the basis of a disability. In the early school years, a child may be found ineligible under the IDEA but eligible under Section 504 and the ADA. The child would then receive services and accommodations under these anti-discrimination laws. In college, the Rehabilitation Act and ADA provide a right to accommodations for qualified persons with disabilities, so that courses, examinations, and activities will be accessible. These laws also require reasonable accommodations in the workplace for qualified individuals with disabilities.

Notice that the protections of these laws are for qualified persons with disabilities. This means you must be qualified to do the college program or job in order to be protected under the law. You may have to prove you are qualified. This is different from public elementary and secondary school, where you were presumed to be qualified to be educated.

An example will illustrate this point. Karen had a reading disorder, auditory processing and memory retrieval problems. She received special education throughout public school. She had extra time on the SAT and did well enough to get into a college social work program. She disclosed her disabilities, requested the accommodation of extra test time and a reader for examinations, and provided supporting professional documentation. She received the requested accommodations but failed essay tests anyway. She was dismissed from the social work program. She then sought to set aside the dismissal on the ground that she couldn't take essay tests on such complex material because of her memory retrieval problem. In the end, the finding was that the school had provided all requested accommodations, that the school had done nothing improper, and that Karen was not qualified for the program.

What Accommodations Would I Be Entitled To In College?

College accommodations depend upon your particular disabilities and how they impact on you in the college setting. Accommodations might include: course accommodations (e.g., taped textbooks, use of a tape recorder, instructions orally and in writing, note taker, and priority seating) and examination accommodations (e.g., extended test time, reader, and quiet room).

What Accommodations Would I Be Entitled To In My Job?

Workplace accommodations depend upon your particular disabilities and how they impact on performing the essential functions of your job. Accommodations might include: instructions orally and in writing, frequent and specific feedback from supervisors, quiet workspace, and training course accommodations.

What About ADHD? Is It Covered Under The Law?

Yes, if it meets the criteria of the particular law. ADHD, while not expressly listed, may be covered by the IDEA under one of three categories: other health impairments, specific LDs, and serious emotional disturbance. ADD has been found to be an impairment under the Rehabilitation Act and ADA and, like LDs, is a disability if it substantially limits a major life activity, such as learning.

How Do I Assert My Rights In College?

You need to disclose your disability to the college, request specific accommodations, and supply supporting professional documentation. In public school, the school system has a duty to identify students with disabilities. This is not so in college. The student has the responsibility to disclose the disability and to request accommodations. You must be specific about the accommodations that you need because of your disability. It is not enough to say that you have LDs, so the college must help you.

Let's look at an example. Sarah is taking courses at the community college. She has a reading disorder, expressive writing disorder, and ADD. She requested one and one-half time on tests, separate room for tests, a reader to read exam questions to her, and a scribe to take down her answers. She provided good professional documentation to support her request and was granted the requested accommodations.

There are student requests that the college is not obligated to grant. For example, if you did not request an accommodation on a test and failed it, generally you may not require the college to eliminate the failure from your record.

Should I Disclose My Disability At Work?

It depends. If you do not need accommodations in the application process; generally it is best to wait until after you have the job. Once on the job, if you see that a part of your job is a problem for you and believe you need an accommodation, it is best to act promptly and not allow a long period of poor performance. Also, at the time you disclose your disability, request the specific reasonable accommodations that will enable you to do your job.

Let's consider an example. Carlos has problems with expressive writing, spelling, and fine motor coordination. After high school, he was hired as a security guard. On the job, he began to have problems with the reports he had to write. The reports were messy, had spelling errors, and were often submitted late. He sensed that his boss was becoming annoyed. Carlos disclosed his disabilities and requested that he be able dictate his reports into his tape recorder and then type them up on one of the computers (with spell check) at the main office at the end of each day. His request was granted.

How Should I Disclose My Disability?

Disclose the disability in writing. Be confident and positive. Combine the disclosure with a request for accommodations that will enable you to perform the job. Provide professional documentation of your disability and need for accommodations.

What Documentation Of My Disability And Need For Accommodations Do I Have To Provide?

You need to provide documentation that establishes that you have a disability and that you need the accommodations you have requested. This might be a letter or report for the college or employer from the professional who has evaluated you. It should state the diagnosis and tests and methods used in the diagnostic process, evaluate how the impairment impacts on you, and recommend reasonable accommodations.

What If I Find Out I Have A Learning Disability During College Or Even Later?

A late diagnosis of LDs may be questioned more than an early diagnosis. It is important to have excellent documentation of the disability. It may be important to explain why the disability was not evident earlier. For example, Janet was diagnosed during her first year of college with a reading disorder. There were reasons why the problem had not shown up earlier. She had done well in the elementary and secondary school because she went to schools that did not have timed tests. She put in the extra time needed to successfully complete her course work and her tests. In college, timed tests posed a major problem for her and led her to seek a thorough evaluation. She was able to document her reading disorder and her need for extra test time in college and medical school.

What If I Take Medication For Attention Deficit Disorder (ADD)? Do I Still Have Rights?

Yes. The existence of a disability is to be judged without reference to the possible beneficial effects of medication. The taking of prescription medication for ADD does not result in loss of disability status under the Rehabilitation Act and ADA or in loss of reasonable accommodations.

Can Learning Disabilities Or ADD Cause A Person To Be Rejected For Service In The Armed Forces?

It depends. Many individuals with LDs or ADD join the Armed Forces and report that the structure and clear expectations help them to do well. However, these conditions may prevent some individuals from obtaining the required score on the Armed Forces Qualifying Test. The Armed Forces are not required to grant accommodations, such as extended test time, on the qualifying test. Further, military regulations provide that academic skills deficits that interfere with school or work after the age of 12 may be a cause for rejection for service in the Armed Forces. These regulations also provide that current use of medication, such as Ritalin or Dexedrine, to improve academic skills is disqualifying for military service.

Can I Be Fired From My Job Or Dismissed From College Even If I Establish That I Have A Disability?

Yes. Having a disability does not create absolute entitlement to a job or college education. The purpose of the anti-discrimination laws is to make sure you have equal opportunity. For example, if you have math disorder and cannot pass a required math course (with no substitutions permitted) for an engineering program, then you would not be qualified for the engineering program.

What About Confidentiality Of Disability Records I File With A College Or An Employer?

Colleges generally have confidentiality policies with respect to disability material. The employment provisions of the ADA contain confidentiality provisions. However, these provisions are not as strong as the IDEA provision that provides for a right to delete disability records contained in your public school files.

For example, Ruth's parents submitted professional documentation of her LDs and depression to her public high school. Ruth submitted the same documentation to her first employer when she disclosed her disabilities and requested job accommodations. After leaving her first job and being hired by a new employer, Ruth decided that she did not need accommodations in the new job. She also decided to request deletion of her disability information from prior files, while retaining copies in her own files in case she would need the records later. The public high school complied with her request. Her first employer informed her that the disability information could not be deleted but was kept in a separate, confidential file.

If I Don't Get What I Ask For, Should I Sue?

A lawsuit is not the first step. First, you must evaluate your own position. It may be wise to consult with a lawyer to review the strong points and weak points in your case. If your case has merit, and you wish to pursue it, then follow these steps: communicate to the college or employer the basic facts and the reasons why you are entitled to what you have requested, negotiate by marshaling the facts that support your request, consider alternative dispute resolution (e.g., mediation and arbitration), and finally consider formal proceedings, such as litigation in the courts.

Remember, even if you have a strong case, it does not mean you must take legal action. You may decide that you wish to put your energy into moving on to a new college program or job rather than disputing events at the prior program.

Part Eight
If You Need More Information

Chapter 58

Directory Of Learning Disabilities Organizations

Government Agencies That Provide Information About Learning Disabilities

Centers for Disease Control and Prevention (CDC)

1600 Clifton Rd.
Atlanta, GA 30329-4027
Toll-Free: 800-CDC-INFO (800-232-4636)
TTY: 888-232-6348
Website: www.cdc.gov
E-mail: CDC-INFO@cdc.gov

Eunice Kennedy Shriver National Institute of Child Health and Human Development (NICHD)

P.O. Box 3006
Rockville, MD 20847
Toll-Free: 800-370-2943
TTY: 888-320-6942
Fax: 866-760-5947
Website: www.nichd.nih.gov
E-mail: NICHDInformationResourceCenter@mail.nih.gov

Resources in this chapter were compiled from several sources deemed reliable; all contact information was verified and updated in January 2017.

National Institute of Neurological Disorders and Stroke (NINDS)

P.O. Box 5801
Bethesda, MD 20824
Toll-Free: 800-352-9424
Phone: 301-496-5751
TTY: 301-468-5981
Website: www.ninds.nih.gov

National Institute on Deafness and Other Communication Disorders (NIDCD)

National Institutes of Health (NIH)
31 Center Dr., MSC 2320
Bethesda, MD 20892-2320
Phone: 301-402-0900
Website: www.nidcd.nih.gov
E-mail: nidcdinfo@nidcd.nih.gov

National Library Service for the Blind and Physically Handicapped (NLS)

Library of Congress (LOC)
1291 Taylor St., N.W.
Washington, DC 20542
Toll Free: 800-424-8567
Phone: 202-707-5100
TDD: 202-707-0744
Fax: 202-707-0712
Website: www.loc.gov/nls
E-mail: nls@loc.gov

Private Agencies That Provide Information About Learning Disabilities

American Speech-Language-Hearing Association (ASHA)

2200 Research Blvd.
Rockville, MD 20850-3289
Toll-Free: 800-638-8255
Phone: 301-296-5700
TTY: 301-296-5650
Fax: 301-296-8580
Website: www.asha.org
E-mail: nsslha@asha.org

Association for Childhood Education International (ACEI)

1200 18th St., N.W.
Ste. 700
Washington, DC 20036
Toll-Free: 800-423-3563
Phone: 202-372-9986
Website: www.acei.org

Autism Society

4340 East-West Hwy
Ste. 350
Bethesda, MD 20814
Toll-Free: 800-3AUTISM (800-328-8476)
Phone: 301-657-0881
Website: www.autism-society.org
E-mail: info@autism-society.org

Center for Parent Information and Resources (CPIR)

35 Halsey St.
4th Fl.
Newark, NJ 07102
Toll Free: 800-695-0285
Website: www.parentcenterhub.org

Charles and Helen Schwab Foundation

201 Mission St.
Ste. 1950
San Francisco, CA 94105
Phone: 415-795-4920
Fax: 415-795-4921
Website: www.schwabfoundation.org
E-mail: info@schwabfoundation.org

Children and Adults with ADD/ADHD (CHADD)

4601 Presidents Dr.
Ste. 300
Lanham, MD 20706
Toll-Free: 800-233-4050
Phone: 301-306-7070
Fax: 301-306-7090
Website: www.chadd.org

Council for Exceptional Children (CEC)

2900 Crystal Dr.
Ste. 1000
Arlington, VA 22202-3557
Toll-Free: 888-232-7733
TTY: 866-915-5000
Website: www.cec.sped.org
E-mail: service@cec.sped.org

Council for Learning Disabilities (CLD)

11184 Antioch Rd.
P.O. Box 405
Overland Park, KS 66210
Phone: 913-491-1011
Fax: 913-491-1011
Website: www.council-for-learning-disabilities.org
E-mail: CLDInfo@cldinternational.org

Division for Learning Disabilities (DLD) of the Council for Exceptional Children (CEC)

Website: www.teachingld.org

Dyspraxia Foundation

84 Westover Rd.
Highwood, IL 60040
Phone: 847-780-3311
Website: www.dyspraxiausa.org

HEATH Resource Center at the National Youth Transitions Center

The George Washington University
2134 G St., N.W.
Washington, DC 20052
Phone: 202-994-1000
Website: www.heath.gwu.edu
E-mail: AskHEATH@gwu.edu

International Dyslexia Association (IDA)

40 York Rd.
4th Fl.
Baltimore, MD 21204
Phone: 410-296-0232
Fax: 410-321-5069
Website: dyslexiaida.org
E-mail: info@dyslexiaida.org

International Dyslexia Association (IDA)

40 York Rd.
4th Fl.
Baltimore, MD 21204
Phone: 410-296-0232
Fax: 410-321-5069
Website: dyslexiaida.org
E-mail: info@dyslexiaida.org

Kaufman Children's Center (KCC)

6625 Daly Rd.
West Bloomfield, MI 48322
Phone: 248-737-3430
Website: kcccloud.com
E-mail: info@kidspeech.com

Learning Ally: Recording for the Blind and Dyslexic (RFB&D)

20 Roszel Rd.
Princeton, NJ 08540
Toll-Free: 800-221-4792
Website: www.learningally.org

Learning Disabilities Association of America (LDA)

4156 Library Rd.
Pittsburgh, PA 15234-1349
Phone: 412-341-1515
Fax: 412-344-0224
Website: ldaamerica.org
E-mail: info@LDAAmerica.org

Learning Disabilities Association of Canada (LDAC)

20 - 2420 Bank St.
Ottawa, Ontario K1V 8S1
Canada
Phone: 613-238-5721
Website: www.ldac-acta.ca
E-mail: info@ldac-acta.ca

Learning Disabilities Association of Newfoundland and Labrador (LDANL)

66 Kenmount Rd.
Ste. 301
St. John's, NL A1B 3V7
Canada
Phone: 709-753-1445
Fax: 709-753-4747
Website: ldanl.ca
E-mail: info@ldanl.ca

Learning Disabilities Worldwide, Inc. (LDW)

14 Nason St.
Maynard, MA 01754
Phone: 978-897-5399
Fax: 978-897-5355
Website: www.ldworldwide.org
E-mail: info@ldworldwide.org

National Aphasia Association (NAA)

P.O. Box 87
Scarsdale, NY 10583
Website: www.aphasia.org
E-mail: naa@aphasia.org

National Association of Special Education Teachers (NASET)

1250 Connecticut Ave., N.W.
Ste. 200
Washington, DC 20036
Toll Free: 800-754-4421
Website: www.naset.org
E-mail: contactus@naset.org

National Center for Learning Disabilities (NCLD)

32 Laight St.
2nd Fl.
New York, NY 10013
Toll Free: 888-575-7373
Phone: 212-545-7510
Fax: 212-545-9665
Website: www.ncld.org

PRO-ED, Inc.

8700 Shoal Creek Blvd.
Austin, TX 78757-6897
Toll-Free: 800-897-3202
Phone: 512-451-3246
Fax: 512-451-8542
Website: www.proedinc.com

Smart Kids with Learning Disabilities

Westport, CT
Website: www.smartkidswithld.org

Chapter 59

Online Apps And Games To Assist With Learning Disabilities

Apps

Easy Spelling Aid
Website: www.easyspellingaid.com

Ghotit Real Writer
Website: www.ghotit.com/dyslexia-software-for-ipad

Lectio
Website: www.mylectio.com

Mystery Word Town
Website: www.artgigapps.com/apps/mystery-word-town

Play & Learn LANGUAGES
Website: www.lyrebirdlearning.com

Promptoo
Website: www.promptoo.com

SightWords
Website: www.sightwords.com/phonemic-awareness

Write in Style
Website: www.gerlingo.com

Resources in this chapter were compiled from several sources deemed reliable; all contact information was verified and updated in January 2017.

Online Games

Anagram Scramble
Website: www.booksandgames.com/freegames/anagram-scramble

Boggle Bash
Website: www.pogo.com/games/boggle-bash

Chicktionary
Website: www.zone.msn.com/en/chicktionary

DefineTime
Website: www.eastoftheweb.com/games/DefineTime1.html

Digging for Answers
Website: www.smithsonianeducation.org/students/ideaLabs/digging_for_answers.html

Frog's Rhyming Machine
Website: www.pbskids.org/wordworld/characters/game_frm.html

Knoword
Website: www.knoword.org

Math Run
Website: www.mathrun.net

Scrabble
Website: www.pogo.com/games/scrabble?pageSection=hp_pop_3scrabble

Text Twist 2
Website: www.wordgames.com/text-twist-2.html

Word Stone
Website: www.wordgames.com/wordstone.html

Word Whomp
Website: www.pogo.com/games/word-whomp?pageSection=hp_pop_4whomp2

Game Websites

Learning Disability Online Game
Website: www.ababasoft.com/games/learning_disability.html

Logic Puzzles
Website: www.puzzles.com/Projects/LogicProblems.html

Index

Index

Page numbers that appear in *Italics* refer to tables or illustrations. Page numbers that have a small 'n' after the page number refer to citation information shown as Notes. Page numbers that appear in **Bold** refer to information contained in boxes within the chapters.

A

ABE *see* adult basic education
abusive head trauma (AHT), overview 151–6
"Abusive Head Trauma (Shaken Baby Syndrome)" (The Nemours Foundation/KidsHealth®) 151n
ACA *see* Patient Protection and Affordable Care Act (2010)
academic instruction, defined 199
academic skills disorders, learning disabilities 34
academics, dyspraxia 72
access technology *see* assistive technology
accommodation
    Americans with Disabilities Act 262
    college transition 279
    dysgraphia 46
    dyslexia 40
    dyspraxia 74
    hidden disabilities 305
    Individualized Education Plan 196
    Individuals with Disabilities Education Act 301
    life skills training 238
    medical examination **311**
    nonverbal learning disability 67
    policy barriers 259
    self-advocacy 253
    transition planning 241

accommodation, *continued*
    workplace 286
    see also college accommodations; job accommodations; public accommodations; reasonable accommodations; testing accommodations
ACE *see* Autism Centers of Excellence
acute lymphoblastic leukemia (ALL), childhood cancer treatment 112
ADA *see* Americans with Disabilities Act
ADA Amendments Act of 2008 *see* Americans with Disabilities Act Amendments Act (ADAAA) of 2008
"ADA Requirements: Testing Accommodations" (DOJ) 229n
ADAAA *see* Americans with Disabilities Act Amendments Act of 2008
adaptive technology *see* assistive technology
ADD *see* attention deficit disorder
adequate yearly progress (AYP), Individuals with Disabilities Education Act 301
ADHD *see* attention deficit hyperactivity disorder
Administration for Children and Families (ACF)
    publication
        epilepsy 127n
adolescents
    attention deficit hyperactivity disorder 89
    learning disabilities diagnosis 23